A Patient's Guide to

Bladder Cancer

Dedicated to patients and caregivers in their pursuit of a cure for bladder cancer

Roswell Park Cancer Institute,
Elm & Carlton Streets,
Buffalo, NY 14263

ISBN-13: 978-1548887407
ISBN-10: 1548887404

TABLE OF CONTENTS

PREFACE

More than a decade of caring for patients with bladder cancer has taught me that they must be actively involved in their own treatment. Bladder cancer is a deadly disease, and successful management demands meticulous attention to detail and careful navigation of complex medical decisions. Keeping patients informed and engaged throughout the process is crucial.

That principle inspired our team to develop a patient-friendly manual aimed at simplifying complicated medical and surgical concepts so that patients and their caregivers can easily understand the processes involved in treating bladder cancer, from diagnosis through recovery. We partnered with experts from all the fields involved in caring for our patients — anesthesiologists, medical oncologists, nurses, ostomy nurses, physical therapists, psychologists, nutritionists and social workers — to address the issues from every angle. I am very proud that the manual we created will serve patients in countries around the globe.

This manual is just one outgrowth of the robot-assisted bladder cancer program at Roswell Park Cancer Institute. Introduced in 2005, it was one of the nation's first formal minimally invasive programs for bladder cancer. Since then, we have performed more than 500 procedures and published landmark articles in the field, both independently and through the International Robotic Cystectomy Consortium. Our work is dedicated to improving care for patients everywhere.

Khurshid A. Guru MD

Chair, Department of Urology

Founded in 1898, Roswell Park was the first research institute in the world to focus exclusively on cancer. Its legacy of discovery and innovation continues today in our mission "to understand, prevent and cure cancer."

Chapter 1

Why Is This Happening To Me?

WHY IS THIS HAPPENING TO ME?

You have been diagnosed with bladder cancer. Getting this news may shock, confuse, and frighten you. Many patients describe the time after diagnosis as an emotional roller coaster. They feel fine one moment and are overwhelmed with emotions the next. You may ask, "Why me?" these are all very normal reactions. When you are ready, talk about it. Not wanting to talk about this right away is also very common.

Although we cannot say for sure why you have this disease, research tells us that many things can increase a person's risk for bladder cancer.

We know that factors such as age, gender, race, and family history may contribute to a person's risk. In addition, smoking and exposure to certain chemicals such as those used in the metal and manufacturing industries can play a role.

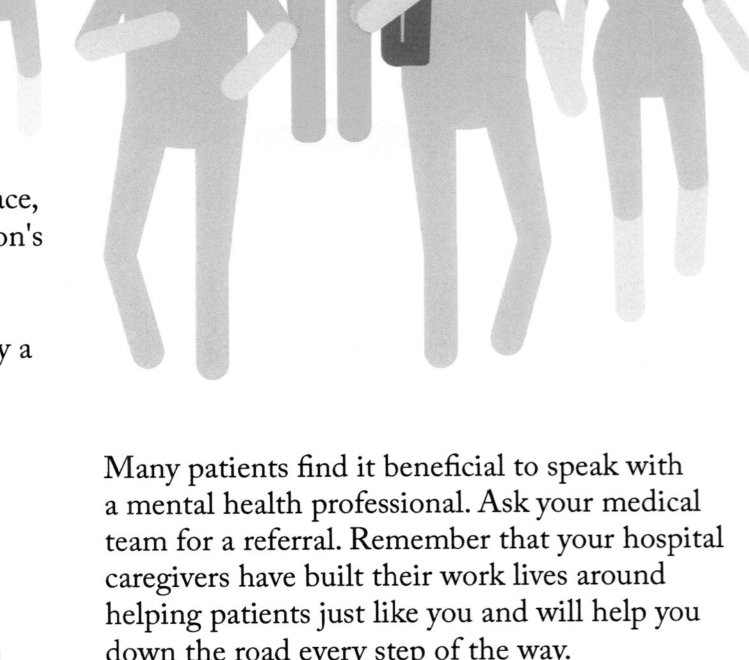

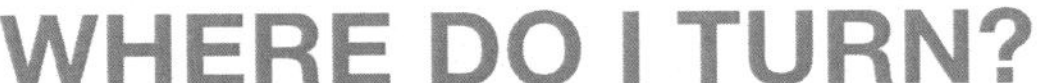

WHERE DO I TURN?

Your Medical Team

Many resources are available to support you and help make life easier. Talk to your medical team about getting help with navigating the healthcare system, as well as social and emotional support for both you and your family members.

Many patients find it beneficial to speak with a mental health professional. Ask your medical team for a referral. Remember that your hospital caregivers have built their work lives around helping patients just like you and will help you down the road every step of the way.

Your Support System

Lean on your family members, friends, and hospital caregivers for support. It is **highly recommended that you bring a close friend or a family member** to your appointments.

It is common to feel overwhelmed by the information you receive. The people who care about you most will also be affected by your diagnosis. Letting them take care of you and talking to them about your feelings and fears can strengthen your relationships and help all of you cope.

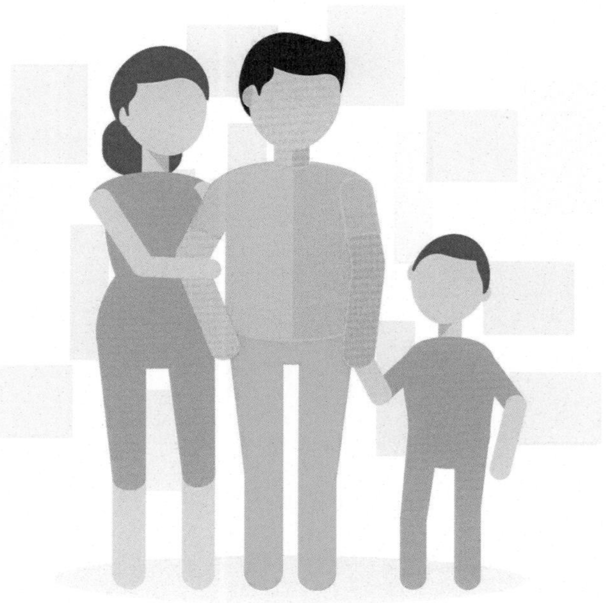

You will likely find that the people you are close to may be supportive in different ways. Some may help with practical matters, such as transportation to appointments or bringing a meal. Others may provide necessary emotional support and be great listeners. And others may help keep your friends and family updated on your progress.

This may be the first time in your life you have had to rely on others and you may feel uncomfortable. Be clear on what you need from these various caregivers so that they know how to be most helpful.

How Do I Take Back Control?

✓ Be Prepared For Medical Appointments

Write down your concerns and questions. This helps ensure that your concerns are addressed and keeps the appointment focused. The more you understand about your condition, the better you will be able to make good decisions.

✓ Ask Questions & Take Notes

Ask if you may record your conversation, or bring a family member or a friend to take notes. It can be very difficult to remember everything, especially while feeling nervous or uncertain.

✓ Gather Information

Gathering appropriate information is important for asking good questions, learning about your cancer, and being your own advocate.

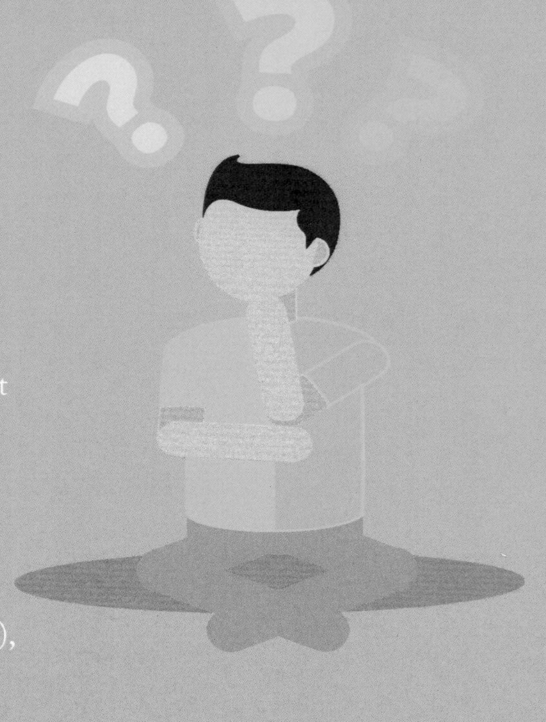

✓ Beware of Misinformation

While the Internet can lead you to a lot of information, there is also a lot of misinformation that may increase anxiety because this information may be false, outdated, or only apply to other patients but not to you.

✓ A good place to start is the National Comprehensive Cancer Network (NCCN) website (https://www.nccn.org), the National Cancer Institute (www.cancer.gov), the American Cancer Society (www.cancer.org), and the Bladder Cancer Advocacy Network (www.bcan.org)

Chapter 2

Going by the Numbers

BLADDER CANCER BY THE NUMBERS

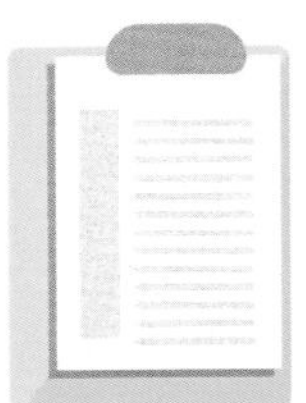

More than
76,000
New Cases
Diagnosed in 2016

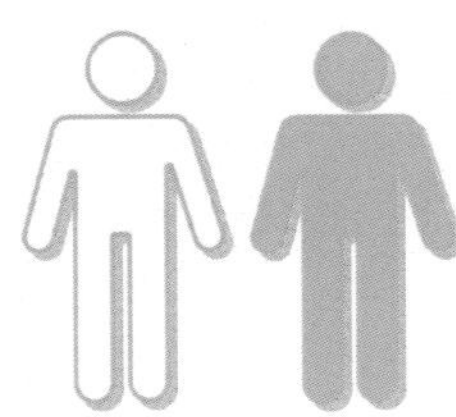

Almost twice as many Caucasian Americans as African-Americans develop bladder cancer. But African – American patients are more likely than Caucasian Americans to have more advanced disease at the time of diagnosis.

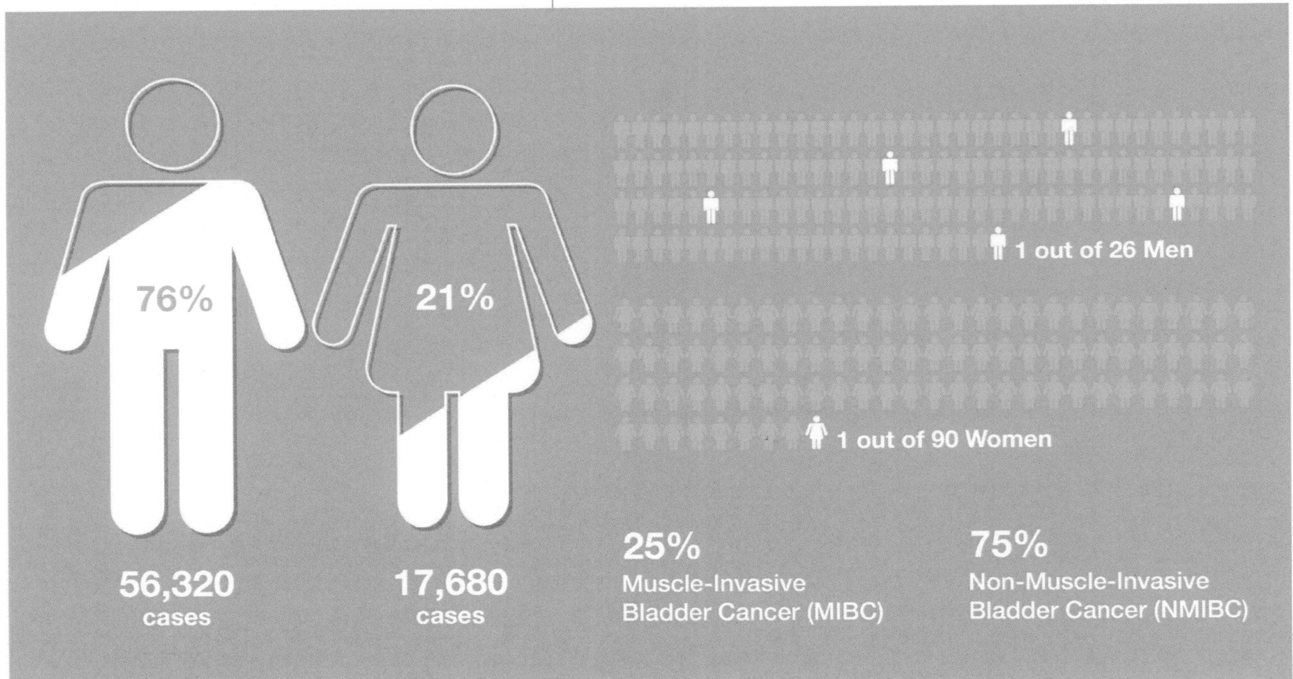

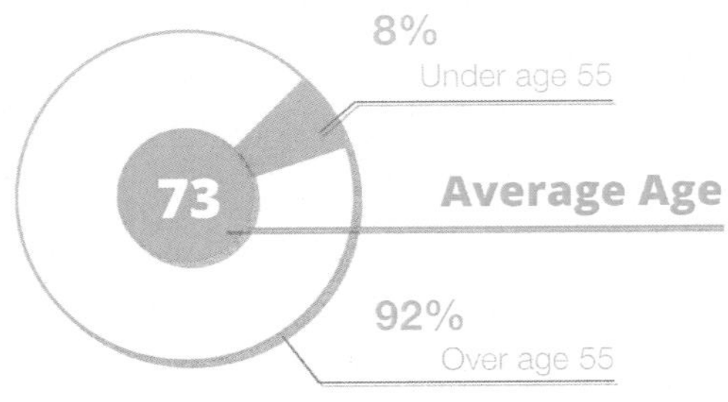

After
5 Years
75% are still alive
In the United States

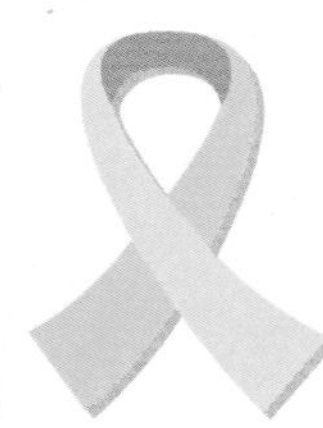

SEER.cancer.org

WHAT ARE THE RISK FACTORS?

Race

Caucasian Americans are most likely to develop bladder cancer. African-Americans tend to have a later stage disease at diagnosis and poorer survival.

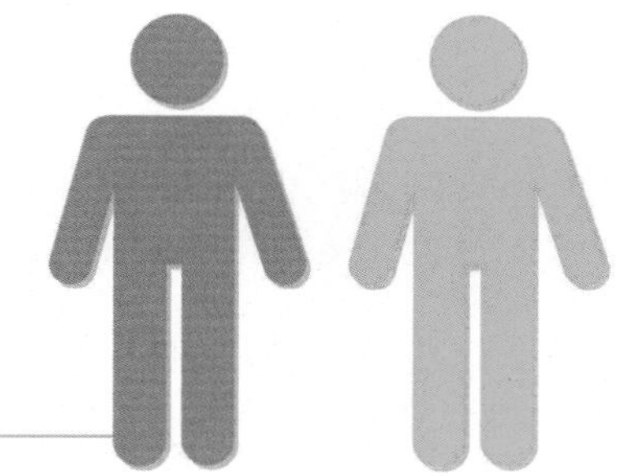

Gender

Men are 3.8 times more likely than women to develop bladder cancer.

Age

Bladder cancer is more frequently diagnosed among people 75-84 years of age. If you are over age 65, you are more likely to develop bladder cancer, and that the tumor will be aggressive.

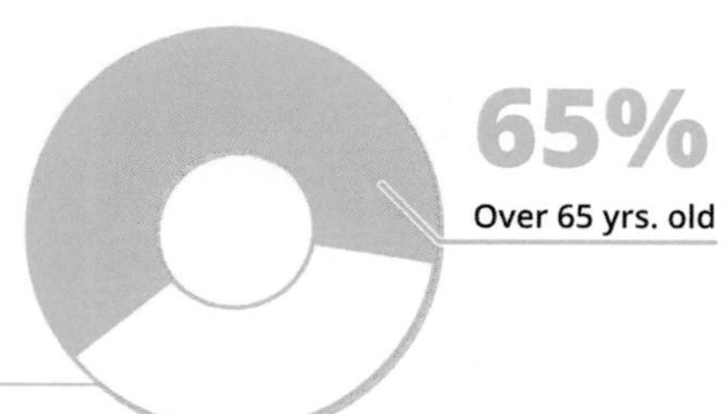

Family History

If you have a first-degree relative (such as a parent, sibling or child) who has had bladder cancer, you are more likely to develop the disease.

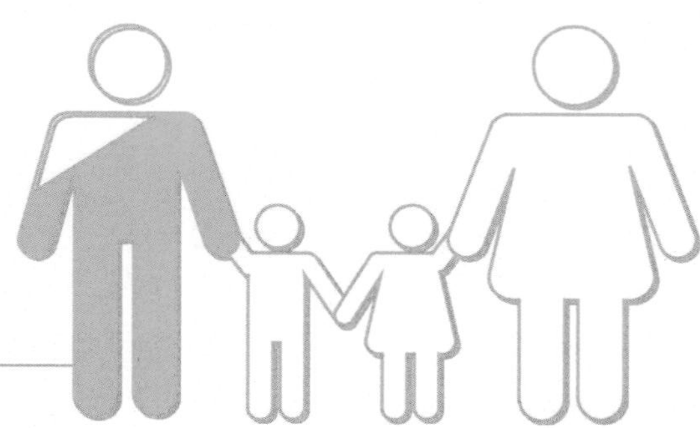

WHICH RISK FACTORS CAN I CONTROL?

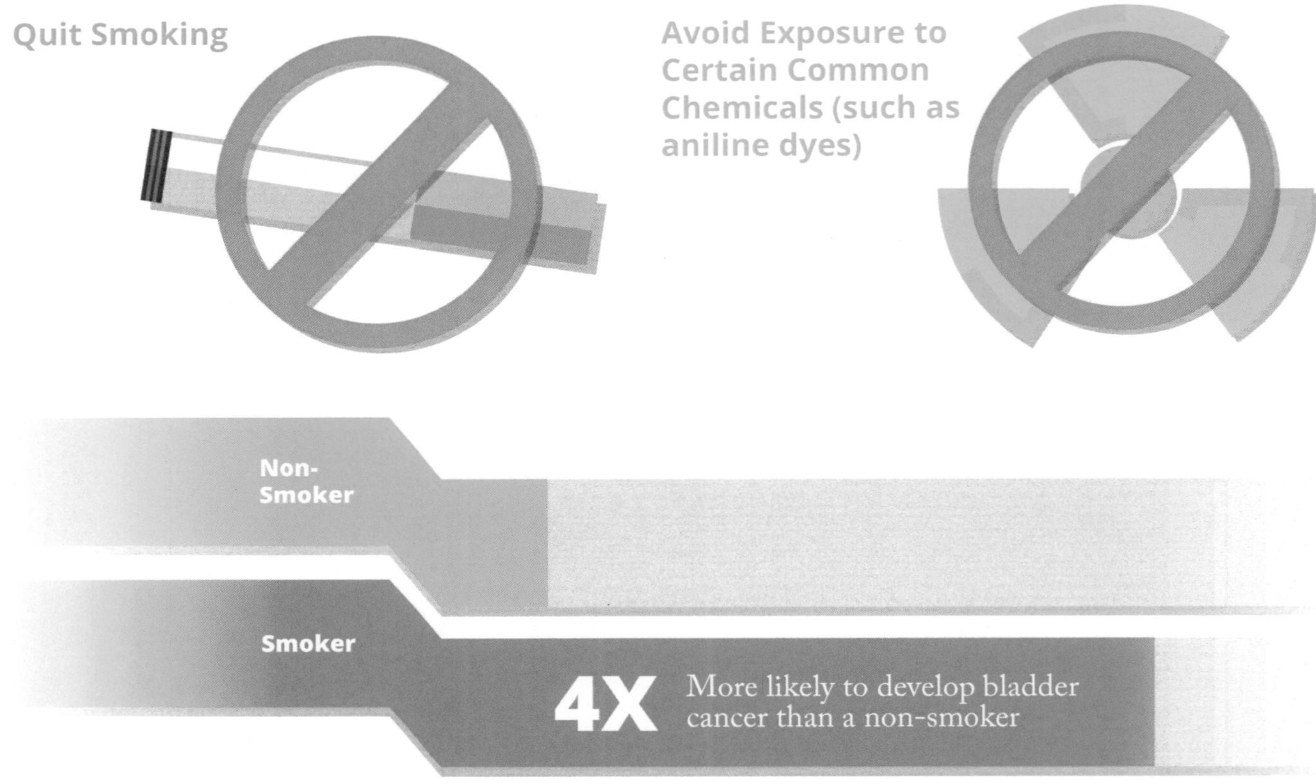

Chemical Exposures

Some occupations have a higher risk of bladder cancer because the work involves exposure to chemicals known to cause cancer. These occupations include:

- ✓ Autoworker
- ✓ Truck driver
- ✓ Barber
- ✓ Metalworker
- ✓ Dry cleaner
- ✓ Painter
- ✓ Paper manufacturer
- ✓ Rope and twine maker
- ✓ Dental technician
- ✓ Drill press operator
- ✓ Apparel manufacturer
- ✓ Machine operator

WHAT ARE MY ODDS?

Survival rates for bladder cancer depend largely on your cancer's stage. Most patients with early-stage disease have a high rate of survival.

Will I Live?

This is the Number One question patients ask when diagnosed with cancer. Survival rates are usually referred to as five-year survival. In other words, how many people with this cancer are still alive five years after their diagnosis? In the United States, the overall five-year survival rate is 75%.

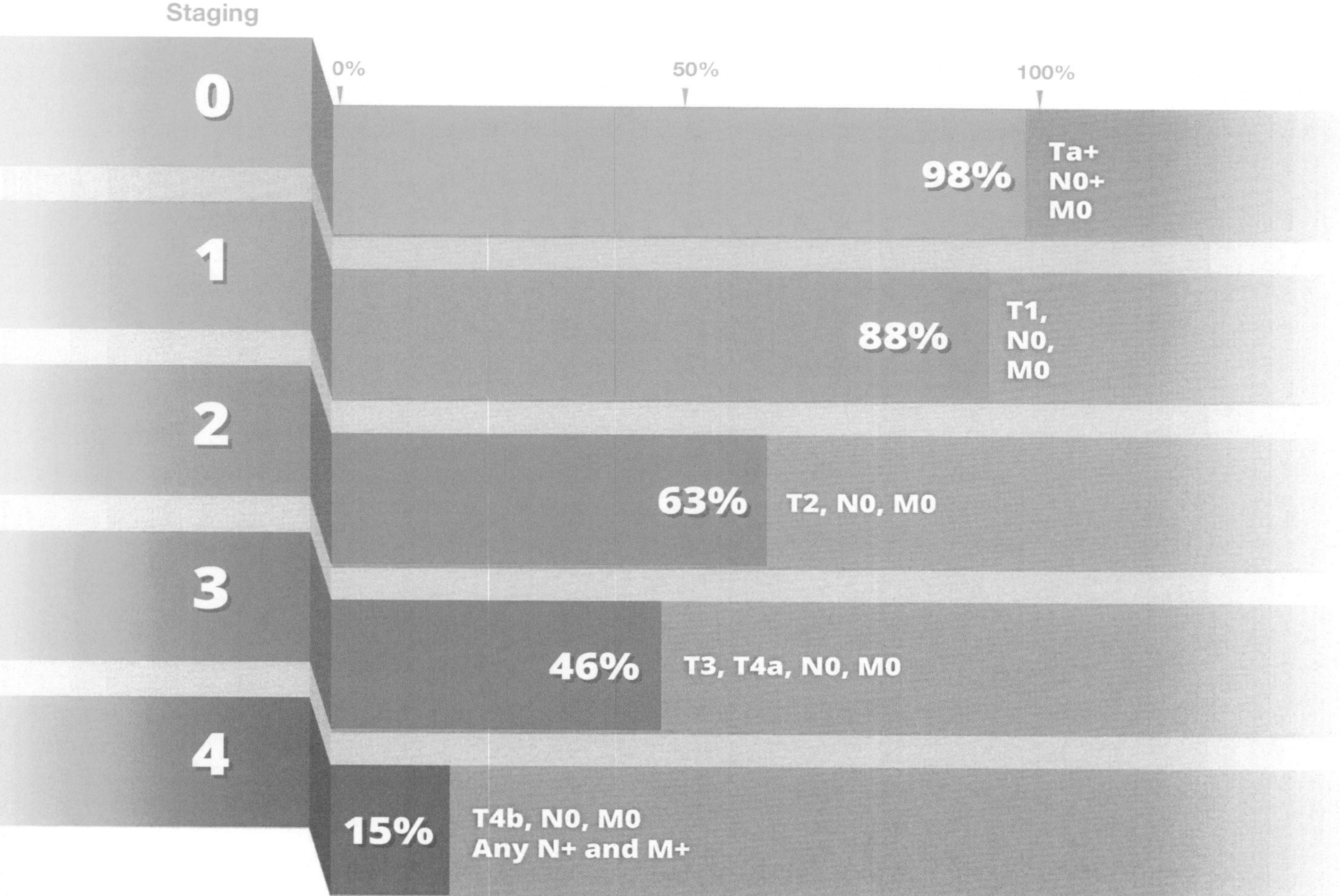

For more information about T-, N- and M-stages please see Chapter 8.

Chapter 3

Your Bladder and Its Neighbors

YOUR BLADDER AND ITS NEIGHBORS

Knowing a little about your anatomy will help you learn where your cancer is located and how it affects your body. Your bladder is part of your urinary system, which is in charge of collecting and ridding of all liquid waste. **Genitourinary system** refers to both the urinary and reproductive systems together. The organs that make up your urinary system are:

Kidneys

The kidneys are located inside your belly, towards your back – one on either side of your backbone (spine). Kidneys remove toxins from your blood and regulate water content by making urine.

Ureters

The ureters are two long tubes that transport urine from the kidneys to the bladder, entering the bladder through openings called ureteric orifices.

Bladder

The bladder is located in the pelvis, between your hip bones. In women, it's in front of the uterus, and in men, it's in front of the rectum. The bladder stores urine until it can be passed out of your body.

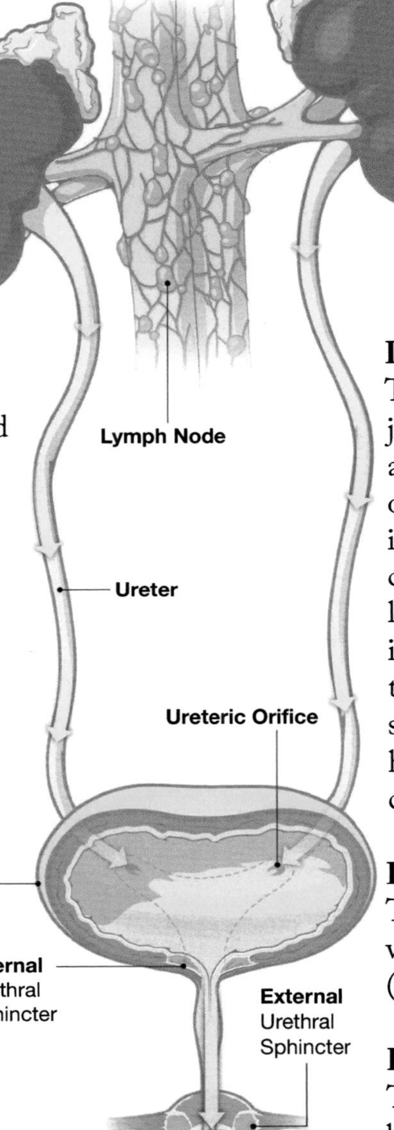

Figure 1.1
Front view of the urinary system

Urethra

The urethra is a small tube that allows urine to travel from the bladder to the outside your body.

Internal sphincter

This sphincter is located at the junction between the bladder and urethra and controls the flow of urine. The internal sphincter is the sphincter that our body controls for us (involuntary). As long as the external sphincter is working properly, you can train your muscles and internal sphincter so that you will not have problems with urine control.

External sphincter

The sphincter that we control when we want to urinate (voluntary).

Lymph Nodes

The lymph nodes are small, lima-bean-shaped tissues within the lymphatic system, a network of hundreds of vessels and nodes, through which lymph fluid travels.

Female Reproductive Organs

Uterus

The uterus, or womb, is a pear-shaped organ in which a fetus grows during pregnancy. The uterus is situated above and behind the bladder. In premenopausal women, the inner layer of the uterus is shed each month during menstruation.

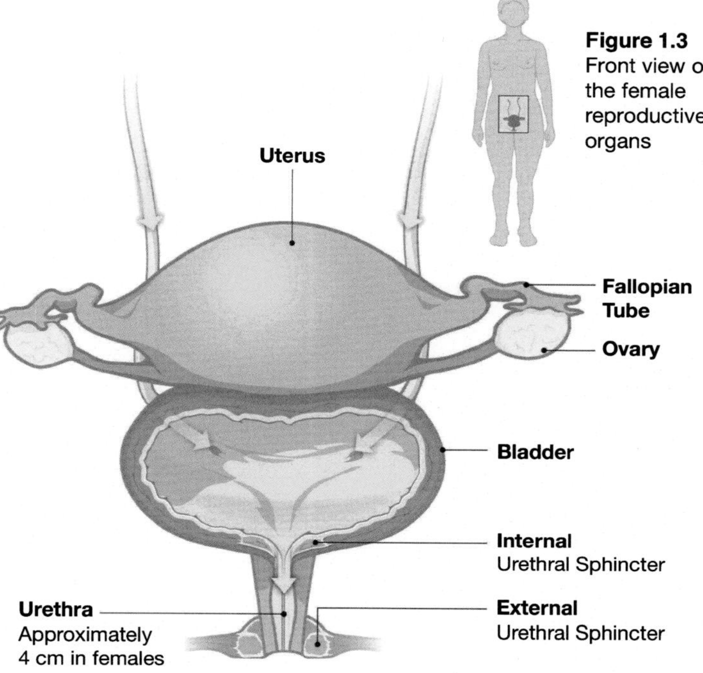

Figure 1.3 Front view of the female reproductive organs

Endometrium

This mucous membrane lining of the uterus thickens during the menstrual cycle in preparation for possible implantation of an embryo.

Ovaries

Women have two ovaries (one on each side of the uterus), each about the size of a large grape. They store and release eggs, and secrete the hormones estrogen and progesterone.

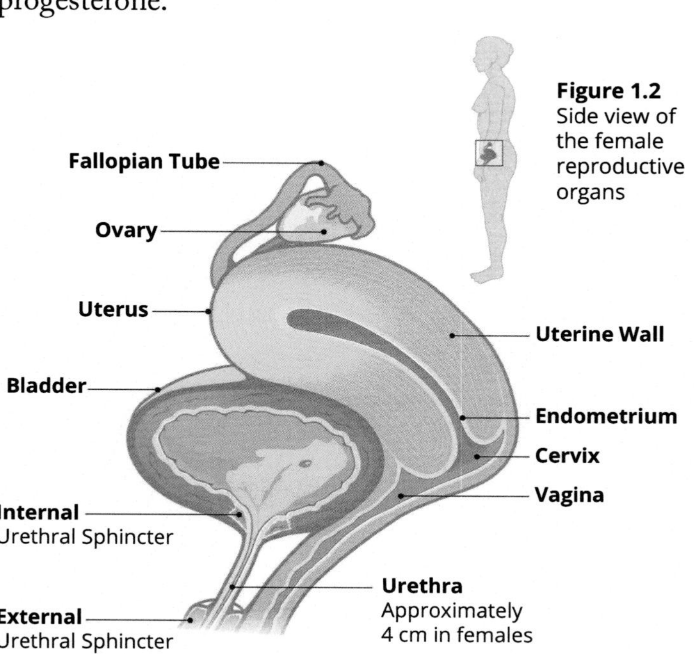

Figure 1.2 Side view of the female reproductive organs

Fallopian Tubes

Women have two fallopian tubes, which connect the uterus to the ovaries. When an egg is released from the ovary, it travels through the fallopian tube to the uterus.

Cervix

The cervix is a cylinder-shaped neck of tissue that connects the vagina and uterus. Located at the lowermost portion of the uterus, the cervix is primarily fibrous, muscular tissue.

Vagina

The vagina is a muscular tube leading from cervix to the external genitals.

Male Reproductive Organs

Testicles (Testes)

Men have two testicles, or testes, which produce sperm and hormones, primarily testosterone.

Prostate

The prostate is a small gland, located below the bladder and completely surrounds the urethra. The prostate gland produces most of the fluid which makes up semen. While not a part of the prostate itself, nerves that control male sexual function travel along the outer capsule of the prostate gland.

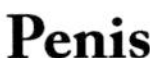

Penis

The penis consists largely of erectile tissue. Urine and semen are discharged from the body through the penis.

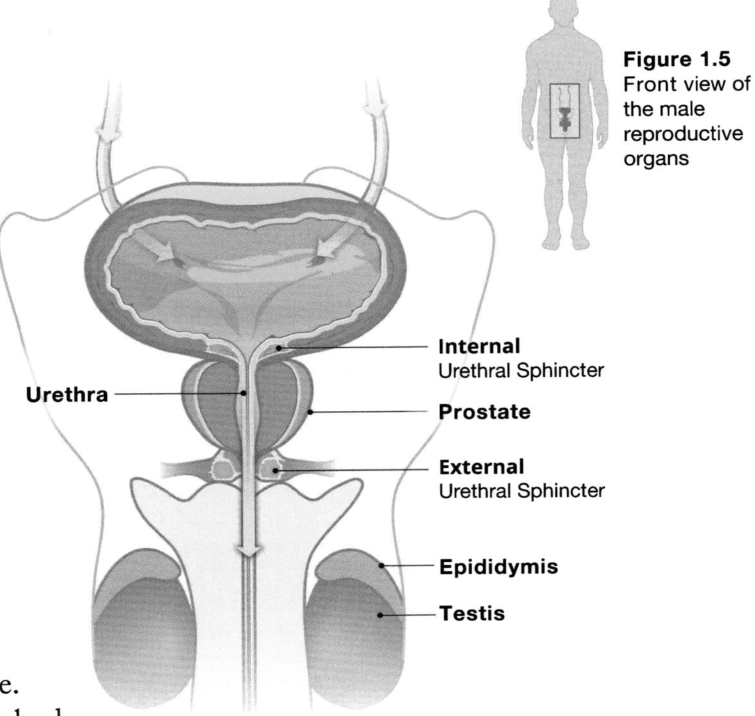

Figure 1.5
Front view of the male reproductive organs

Figure 1.4
Side view of the male reproductive organs

Seminal Vesicles

The seminal vesicles, also known as the seminal glands, are a pair of simple tubular glands located within the pelvis behind the male urinary bladder. They also secrete fluid that makes up semen.

Chapter 4

Confirming Your Diagnosis With Cystoscopy

FLEXIBLE CYSTOSCOPY

Flexible cystoscopy is a procedure which allows your doctor to see the inside of your bladder. A tube called a cystoscope is passed into your bladder. The cystoscope has a light and a camera at the end of it so your doctor can better visualize the inside of your bladder. This procedure can be done in your doctor's office.

Why Do I Need a Cystoscopy?

Several reasons why you may need a cystoscopy:

- You have visible blood in your urine.
- A urine test showed microscopic blood in your urine (that you cannot see with your naked eye).
- You have symptoms such as frequency or urgency of urination

This test allows your doctor to collect cells from the lining of your bladder to examine, diagnose and treat various bladder conditions. Your doctor may also perform a bladder wash during cystoscopy.

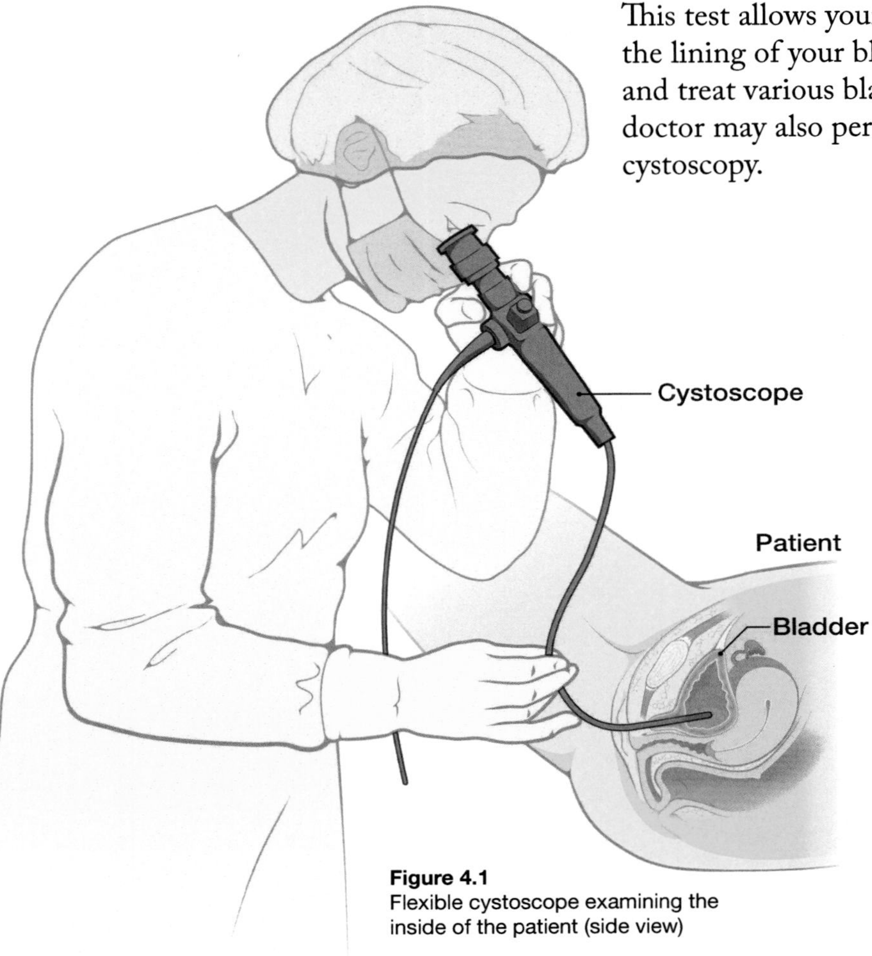

Figure 4.1
Flexible cystoscope examining the inside of the patient (side view)

What to Expect

1 Waiting Room to Procedure Room

- Undress from waist down.
- Position your back on the exam table. (Procedure can also be performed in wheelchair.)
- Raise your knees and spread them apart.

2 Preparation

- A nurse will clean the area around your urethra with a cold solution to help eliminate bacteria.
- Then a clear numbing gel is inserted into the urethra. It will take a few minutes for it to take effect.
(You may feel a slight burning or pressure when gel is inserted.)

3 Procedure

- Doctor will gently advance cystoscope through urethra into bladder.
- Occasionally, the area around the sphincter is difficult to pass. Your doctor may ask you to take a deep breath while passing across this resistance.
- A solution will flow into the bladder to stretch and distend the bladder.
(You may feel the urge to urinate as your bladder fills. If you wish, ask your doctor if you may view the procedure on the monitor.)

4 End of Procedure

- Once the examination is finished, the cystoscope is removed.
- You should urinate before leaving the office.
(Entire procedure takes about 15-30 minutes.)

What is the Doctor Looking for Inside My Bladder?

Your doctor will look for any abnormalities in the urethra and the lining of your entire bladder, such as:

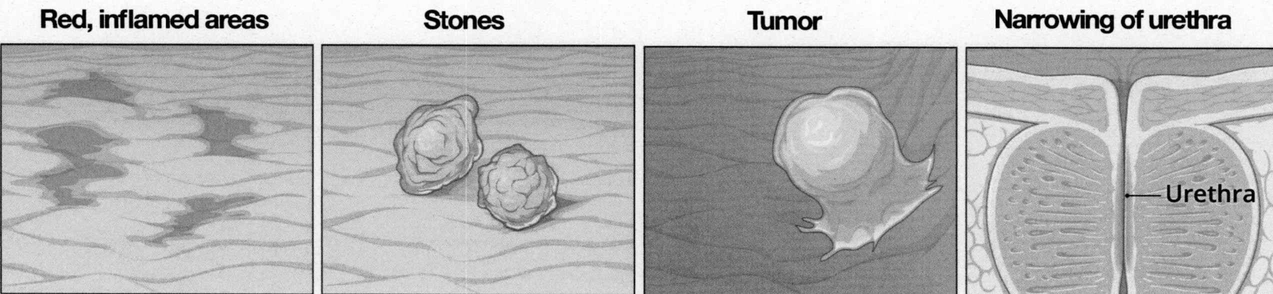

Figure 4.2
Abnormalities

What Can I Expect After the Procedure?

You will most likely experience a burning sensation when you urinate, but this should go away quickly. You may see small amounts of blood in your urine, or have the urge to urinate more frequently.

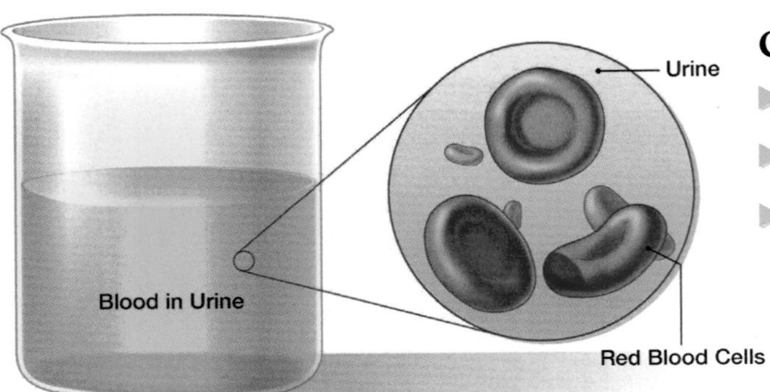

Figure 4.3
Urine mixed with blood

What Should I Know?

- Increase your fluid intake for the first few hours after the procedure.
- Rarely, some patients develop a urinary tract infection after cystoscopy. To prevent this, your doctor may prescribe an antibiotic.

When Should I Call My Doctor?

Call your doctor immediately if you:

- Experience excessive bleeding
- Cannot urinate
- Have chills, fever or pain

Chapter 5

Has My Cancer Spread?

HAS MY CANCER SPREAD?

In order to determine whether or not your cancer has spread beyond your bladder, your medical team will order one or more imaging scans to get a better picture of your disease. Imaging tests such as CT, MRI, PET and bone scans are most commonly used for patients with bladder cancer. These scans may be inconvenient but are painless. Some patients feel discomfort from an injection, or feel anxiety from being in a small space.

Computerized Tomography (CT)

Computerized tomography (CT), also known as computerized axial tomography (CAT scan) uses x-rays to capture three-dimensional (3D) images of certain areas of your body and depicts bones, organs, and other tissues.

Figure 5.1
CT scan of the pelvis with IV contrast showing a bladder mass

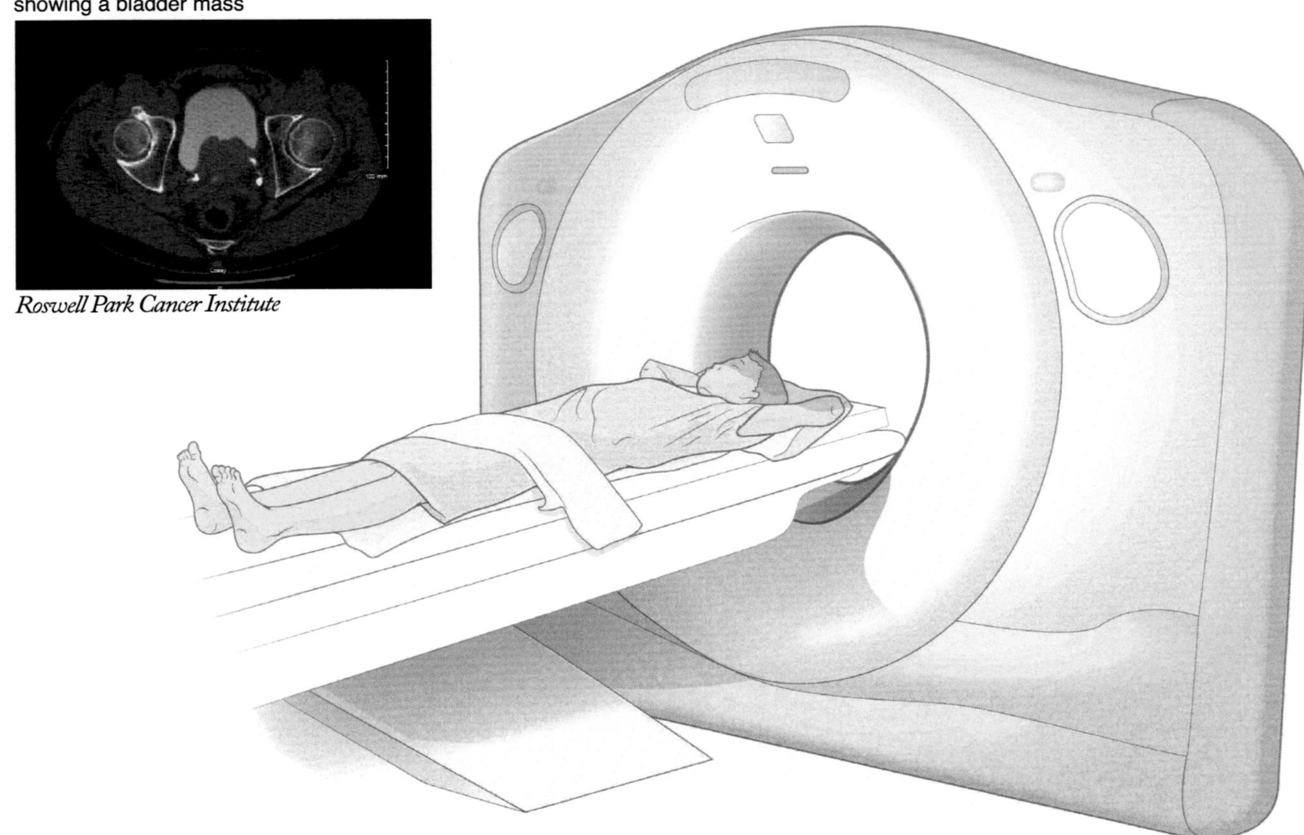

Roswell Park Cancer Institute

Figure 5.2
A typical computerized tomography (CT) machine

Magnetic Resonance Imaging (MRI)

Magnetic Resonance Imaging scans (MRIs) are similar to CT scans, but instead of x-rays, MRIs use magnetic fields and pulses of radio waves to take pictures of your body. MRIs can be safer because they do not expose you to radiation. However, MRI is more expensive than other scans and take longer (between 30 minutes and two hours). The MRI machine has a smaller opening for your body than the CT machine, which may feel constricting or be more difficult for a larger person.

Figure 5.4
MRI of a male pelvis (axial view)

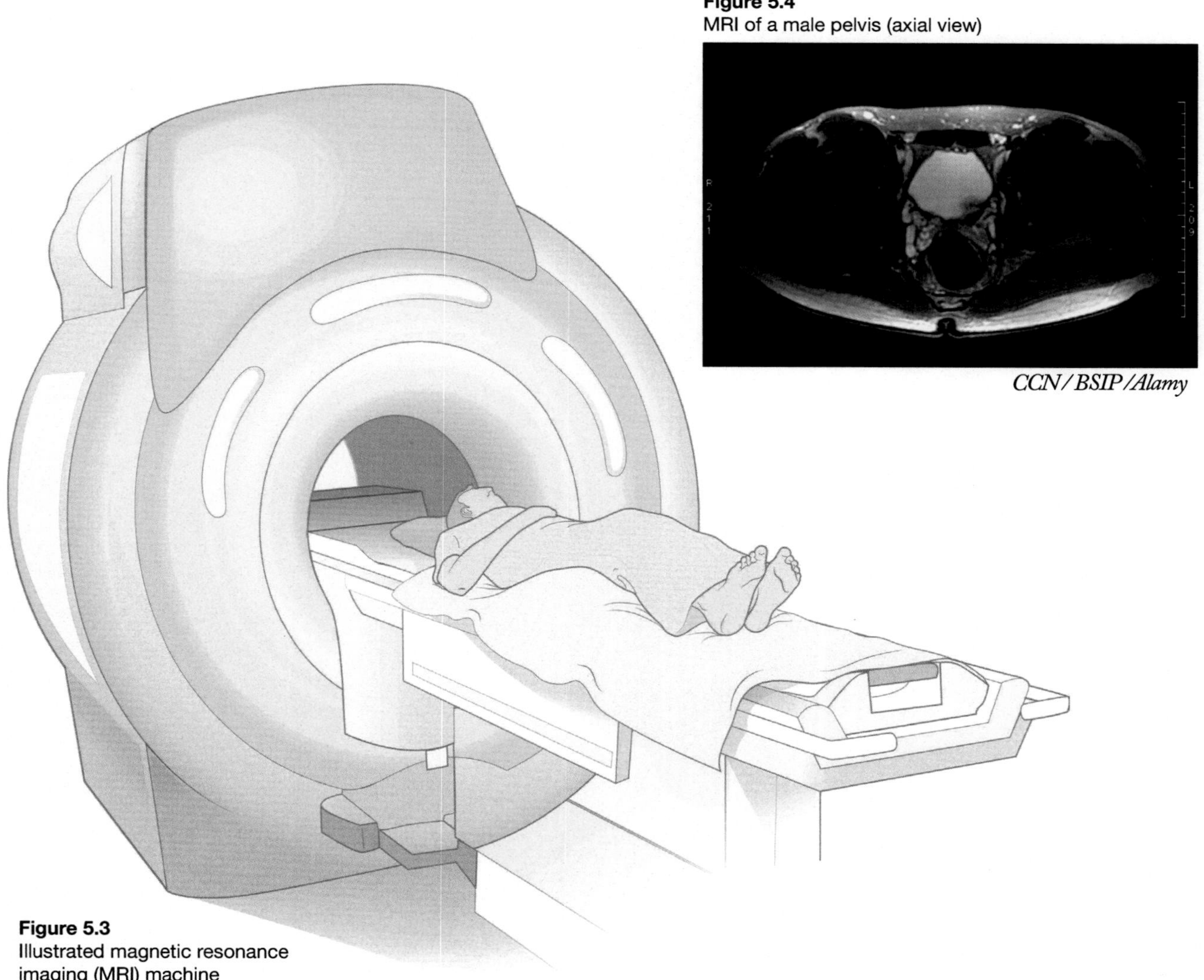

CCN/BSIP/Alamy

Figure 5.3
Illustrated magnetic resonance imaging (MRI) machine

Positron Emission Tomography (PET)

Positron Emission Tomography (PET) scans take images of your body after a tiny amount of radioactive material called a tracer is injected. PET scans may help detect disease earlier than other scans. PET and PET/CT scans can be used for cancer detection and staging (determining whether cancer has spread in the body).

How is PET different from CTs and MRIs?

PET scans are better at showing your body's processes. They look at the metabolism of your tissues as well as your anatomy. This may make them more sensitive and specific, differentiating normal benign cells from highly-metabolically-active cancer cells.

During the scan, an area where a lot of tracer sticks is called a "hot spot", or more active area of your body. An area where very little tracer sticks is called a "cold spot" or less active area of your body. A hot spot does not mean that the area has cancer but that it may need a closer look.

Figure 5.5
An example of a PET scan image

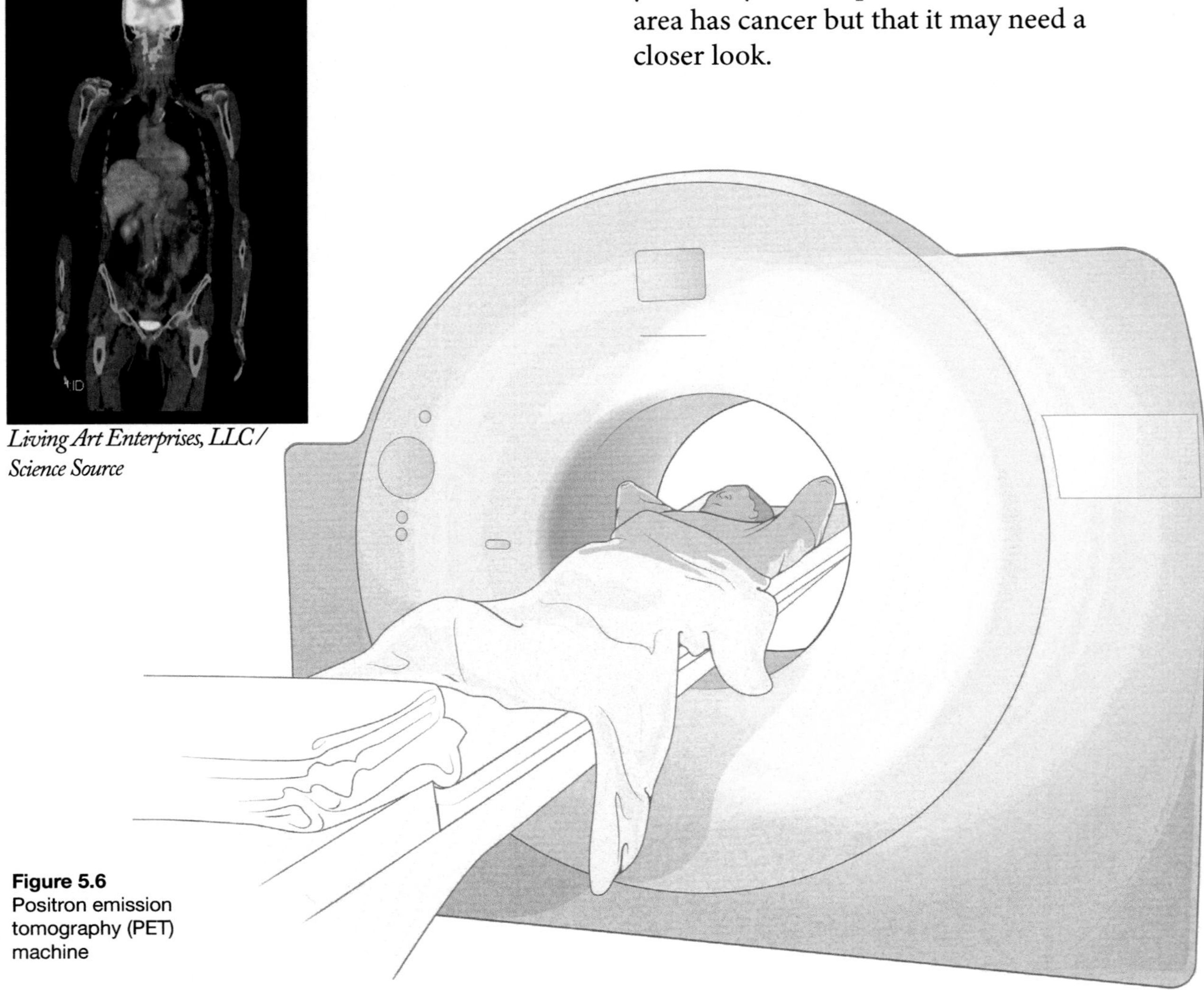

Living Art Enterprises, LLC / Science Source

Figure 5.6
Positron emission tomography (PET) machine

Bone Scan

A bone scan can determine if this is cancer whether your cancer has spread into your bones. Bone scans also use a radioactive tracer injected into your veins in different areas of your body.

Once the tracer is injected, your medical team may want to start a scan right away or wait until the tracer has started to move deeper into your bones, which can take between two and four hours. You will need to drink plenty of water after the tracer is injected to help wash out any remaining tracer that does not go into your bones. You should urinate out the rest of the tracer from your body before your scan. The actual scan will take about one hour. It usually examines your whole body.

Figure 5.8
An example of a bone scan image

Scott Camazine / Science Source

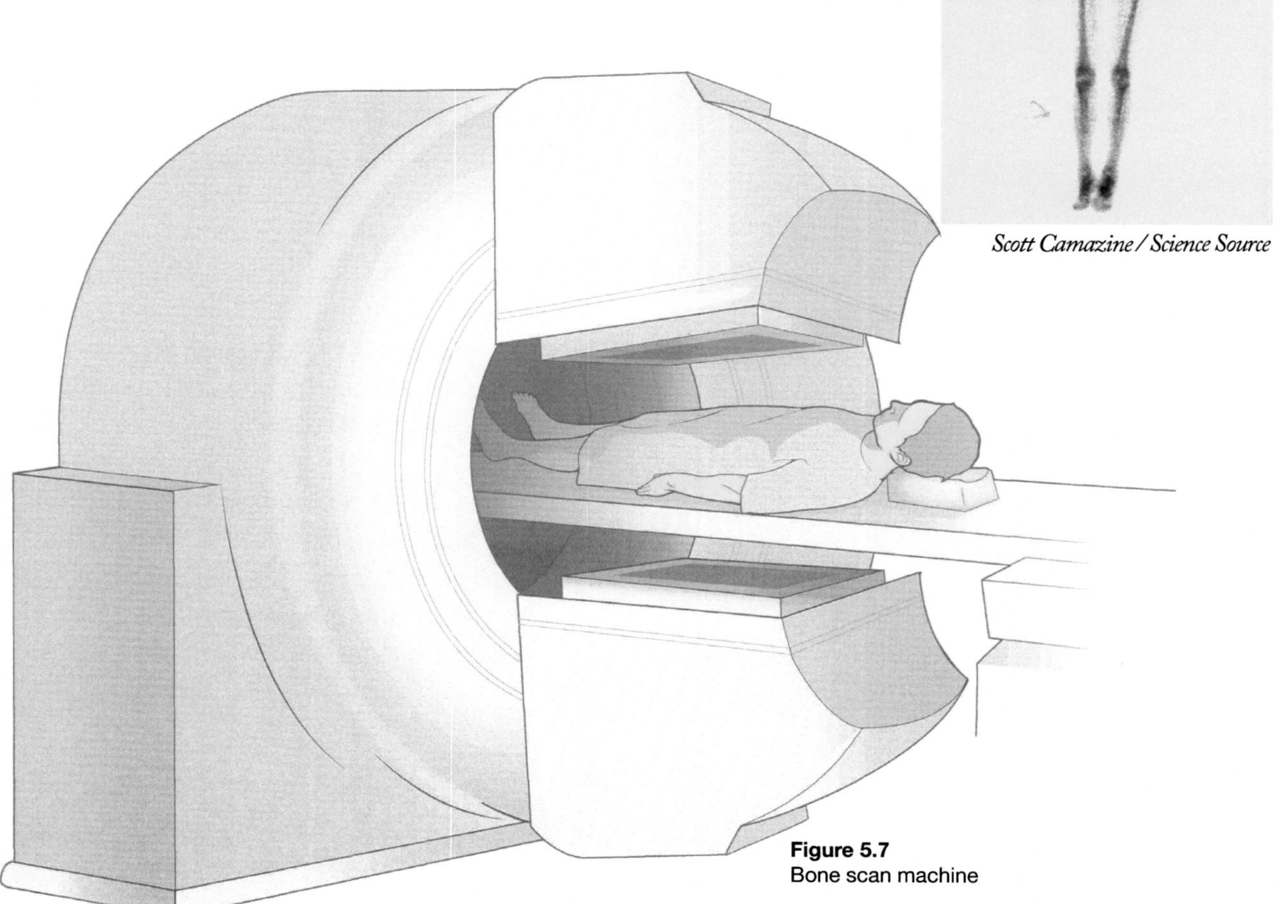

Figure 5.7
Bone scan machine

Scan	Time It Takes	Benefits/Limitations
CT	15 min - 1 hour	- Exposure to x-rays - Allergy to contrast dye can be toxic to kidneys
MRI	30 min - 2 hours	- No exposure to x-rays - Contrast tracer can be toxic to kidneys - May not be used in people with pacemakers; - Some people are uncomfortable in small spaces
PET	2 - 5 hours (tracer & scan)	- Moderate exposure to x-rays - Radioactive material (tracer) required
Bone Scan	2 - 5 hours (tracer & scan)	- Moderate exposure to x-rays

Before Scans

Before your scan, tell your medical team if you:

- Have any allergies (seafood, iodine, or other allergies)
- Have had a bad reaction to scans in the past, or are taking any medications, vitamins, or herbal supplements
- Are breastfeeding
- May be pregnant
- Have any metal in your body (cardiac pacemaker, brain aneurysm clips, pins, plates, metal rods, etc.)
- Have a history of kidney disease or diabetes
- Are claustrophobic (have fear of tight spaces) or have asthma or anxiety problems
- Will have a hard time lying still on your back for 30 minutes to four hours

What Will Happen?

You will be given a hospital gown to change into. Be sure to remove all clothing and metal objects, including hearing aids and removable dental work. Credit cards or any other magnetic scanning strips should NOT be brought into the exam room, because the scanner may break them. If you have any metal in your body, you should not have certain scans.

You may be instructed to drink plenty of water and visit the restroom to urinate before your scan. Or you may need to avoid eating or drinking certain things before your scan. Follow your medical team's instructions carefully so that you won't need to repeat the scan.

Contrast (CT/MRI)

In order to provide clearer images of a specific area, the physician may recommend a chemical dye known as "contrast" that is picked up by the scanner. Contrast is not used as often in MRIs as it is in CT scans.

The contrast can be administered various ways:

1. Orally: swallowed in a liquid
2. Intravenously: inserted into your veins through a needle
3. Enema: a liquid flushed into your rectum
4. Gaseous: inhaled into the lungs (rare, but not painful)

The way the contrast is delivered will depend on where your disease is in your body.

Contrast Symptoms:

- Feeling flushed
- Metallic taste
- Feeling as though you are peeing
- Slight burning

Contrast Side Effects:

- Shortness of breath; wheezing
- Nausea
- Itching/Facial swelling
- Rash

Tracer (PET/Bone)

For PET or bone scans, a radioactive tracer may be injected into your veins in different areas of your body. The tracer should not cause any symptoms or side effects unless you have an allergic reaction or have diabetes. There should be no tracer left in your body 48 hours after injection.

Tracer Side Effects:

- Shortness of breath; wheezing
- Nausea

Figure 5.9
Medical professional injecting radioactive space tracer

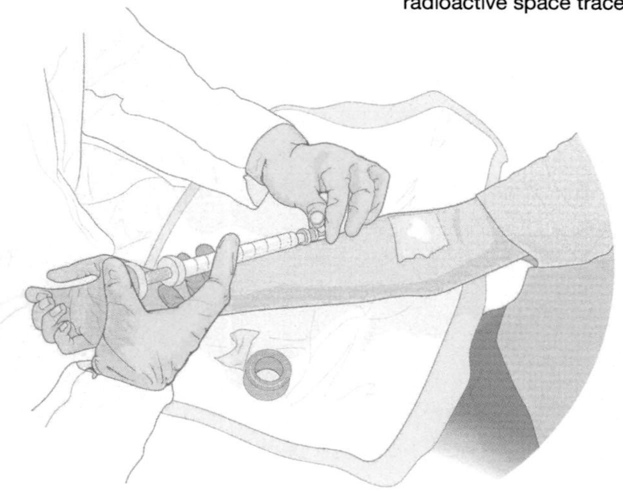

- Itching/facial swelling
- Rash
- Abnormalities in blood sugar or insulin levels

During the Scan

You will be brought into the room where the scan will be performed and asked to lie down on a narrow table. The team will slide you through the center opening of the scanner. If you have an IV, this may be attached to a bag of contrast before the scan begins.

When the scan begins, the machine will rotate around your body slowly. The machine will make a loud whirring noise and you may feel a little constricted, but the machine will not touch you. Alert your medical team beforehand if you are anxious about being in this small space (claustrophobic). It is important to stay as still as possible during your scan. Moving may make the picture blurry and require you to repeat the scan.

After the Scan

You should be able to go about your normal activities unless your medical team tells you otherwise. Any radioactive material that your body has taken in won't endanger you or the people around you, and it should be completely gone from your body within 48 hours. Continue to drink plenty of water to flush the material out of your body quicker.

Your medical team will look carefully at the pictures from your scan for signs of cancer. Depending on what they learned from your scan, your medical team may do more tests to confirm their findings.

Biopsy and Scan

Although scans can provide your medical team with a picture of your body's structure and function, scans cannot tell what is going on in your cells. A scan may direct your medical team to an area of your body that requires a closer look.

A biopsy removes a tiny piece of tissue from your body to look for disease. By carefully examining a biopsy, your medical team may find cancer cells or no cancer cells. Taking a biopsy is usually an invasive process to reach the area in question and take out some tissue.

Chapter 6

Getting a Biopsy: Transurethral Surgery

TRANSURETHRAL SURGERY

Figure 6.1
Transurethral resection of bladder tumor using a resectoscope

In order to identify the nature, type, size and depth of your cancer, your doctor will need a biopsy or tissue sample of the tumor or lesion to send to a pathology laboratory. In order to obtain this biopsy, your doctor will perform a procedure called a Transurethral Resection of Bladder Tumor (TURBT). If your cystoscopy or an imaging scan found a suspicious mass or any irregularity (lesion), you will most likely need a TURBT.

TURBT is essential to obtain a biopsy to confirm the cancer diagnosis and determine the stage and grade of your cancer. This will also help determine the type of treatment best suited for you.

This procedure may remove a piece of tumor tissue, or the entire tumor, from the bladder. The tumor tissue is sent to a pathology laboratory for examination under a microscope. (Learn more about pathology in the next chapter).

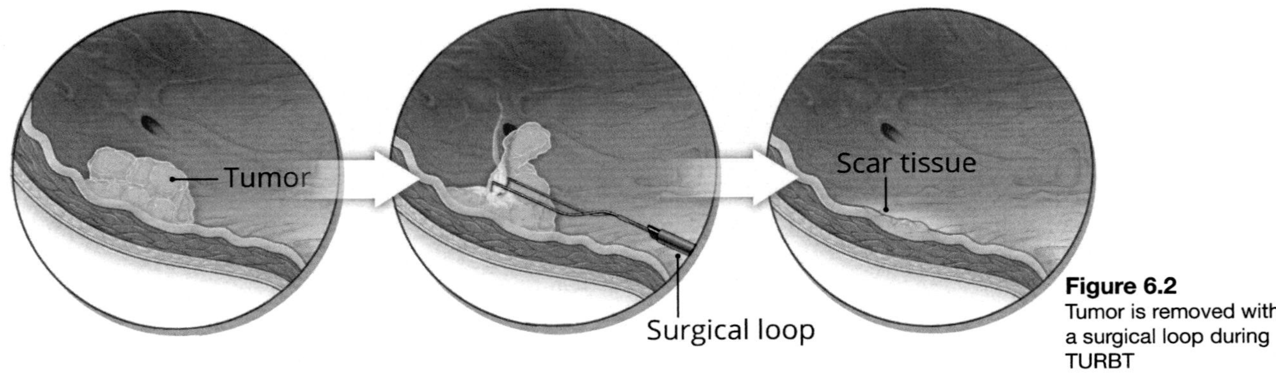

Figure 6.2
Tumor is removed with a surgical loop during TURBT

What Happens During the Surgery?

At the start of the procedure, you will be given a numbing drug (anesthetic). Generally, two options are available: 1) general anesthesia, where you take a nap for the entire procedure, or 2) local anesthesia where you stay awake and after being given a drug through a needle in your lower back to numb the lower half of your body.

What Happens After the TURBT Surgery?

You will either go home the same day or stay in the hospital overnight. For a few days you may wear a small drainage tube, called a catheter, to help drain your urine. After the surgery, you may have some bleeding and pain when passing urine. You may also have to urinate more often. These side effects should go away within two weeks of the operation.

If you have bleeding after TURBT, please use Figure 7.5 in chapter 7 to describe how much bleeding you have to the physician. If you have pain, your physician can give you medication to relax your bladder and avoid spasms.

Intravesical Chemotherapy

Some patients have chemotherapy treatments in which the drug is injected directly into the bladder through the catheter called Intravesical Chemotherapy, this treatment is used mainly after transurethral resection of bladder tumors.

The drug (most commonly mitomycin C) fills the bladder and destroys any remaining tumor cells not removed by the process. If the tumor is more solid or the surgery was extensive, chemotherapy may not be given.

Do I Need the TURBT Surgery Again?

Based on the results of your TURBT and your cancer's stage, your medical team will decide how to move forward.

- You will need to have your bladder checked at regular intervals, depending on your disease risk.
- You may need to have more frequent checkups if you are at higher risk.

Chapter 7

Caring for the Foley Catheter

CARING FOR THE FOLEY CATHETER

You may need a Foley catheter to drain your bladder following TURBT, to allow your bladder to heal.

What is a Foley Catheter?

A Foley catheter is a soft plastic tube that is inserted into the bladder to drain your urine into an attached collection bag. A small balloon at one end of the catheter keeps it in place in your bladder.

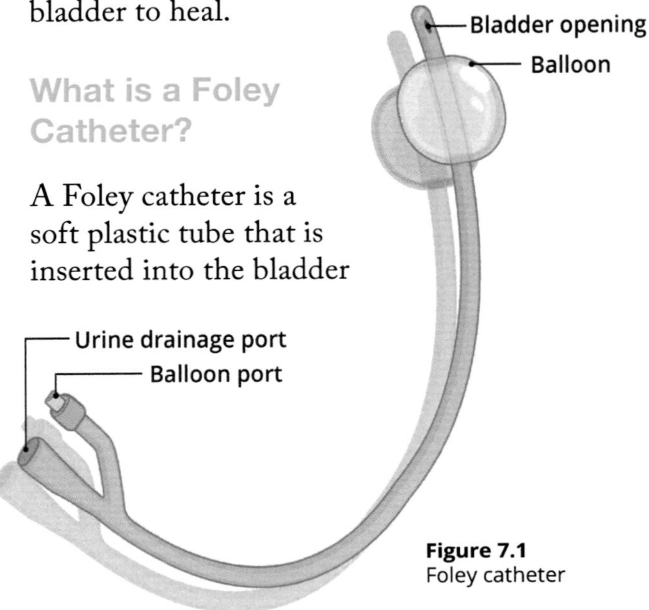

Figure 7.1
Foley catheter

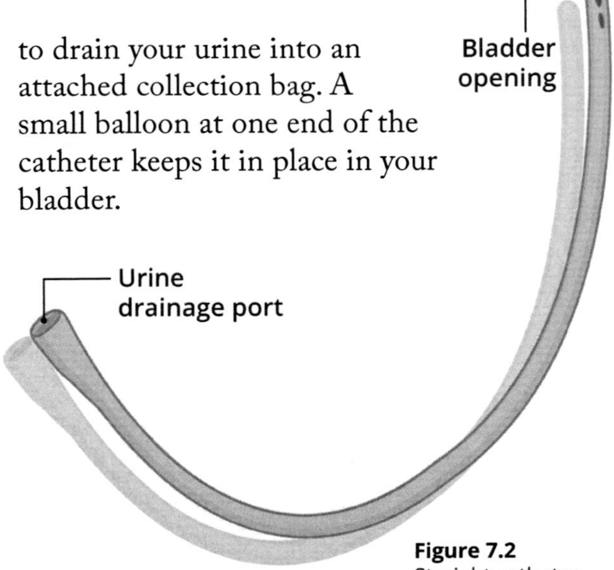

Figure 7.2
Straight catheter

What is a Straight Catheter?

This catheter type is used only for draining and irrigation. It does not have a balloon at the end and does not remain in your body.

How to Care for Your Catheter

Caring for your catheter is important to prevent infection and promote healing. You must cleanse the urethral area (where the catheter exits the body) and the catheter itself with soap and water daily. You should follow these care tips:

- Increase your fluid intake (especially water) unless you are on fluid restrictions.
- Cleanse yourself thoroughly after all bowel movements.
- Wash your hands before and after handling the catheter. Do not allow the outlet (urine drainage port shown on Figure 7.1) to touch anything. If the outlet is unclean, it should be cleaned with soap and water.
- Men may notice pink-colored mucus discharge at the tip of their penis. This is a normal reaction to the urethral irritation from the catheter.
- To reduce this irritation, apply water-based lubricant ointment around the tip of the penis, where the catheter enters, up to four times a day.
- Keep the drainage bag below your waist so it remains lower than the bladder and prevents urine from flowing back up into your bladder.
- Empty the collection bag at least every six hours or when 3/4 full.

- Ask for a night bag and a leg bag so you will be able to move around.

How to Clean the Drainage Bag

- Remove the drainage bag from the catheter and attach the catheter to a second bag during the cleaning.
- Rinse the bag with warm soapy water.
- Hang the bag with the outlet valve open to allow it to drain and dry.

Some Issues With the Foley Catheter

Leaking

If you have urine leaking around the catheter where it enters your urethra, the catheter may be blocked or you may be experiencing bladder spasms. If this is due to blockage, you may have abdominal pain, no urine, or blood clots in urine. Irrigating your bladder may help stop the leaking.

Bladder spasms

You may experience bladder spasms while the catheter is in the bladder. You may feel pain in the tip of your penis, and/or pain in your lower abdominal or pelvic area and urinary or bloody discharge around the catheter's insertion site. To minimize spasms use stool softeners to avoid constipation and avoid any sudden movements that may pull on the catheter. If spasms become severe or painful, your doctor can prescribe medication to ease them.

Swelling or bruising

Men may find that their scrotum and penile area may become swollen or bruised for a day or two after surgery. This is normal and should go away after the catheter is removed. To help reduce swelling, place a rolled-up towel underneath the scrotum whenever you are sitting or lying down.

Blood clots in your urine

Small blood clots are normal and will go away on their own. Large clots, however, can block

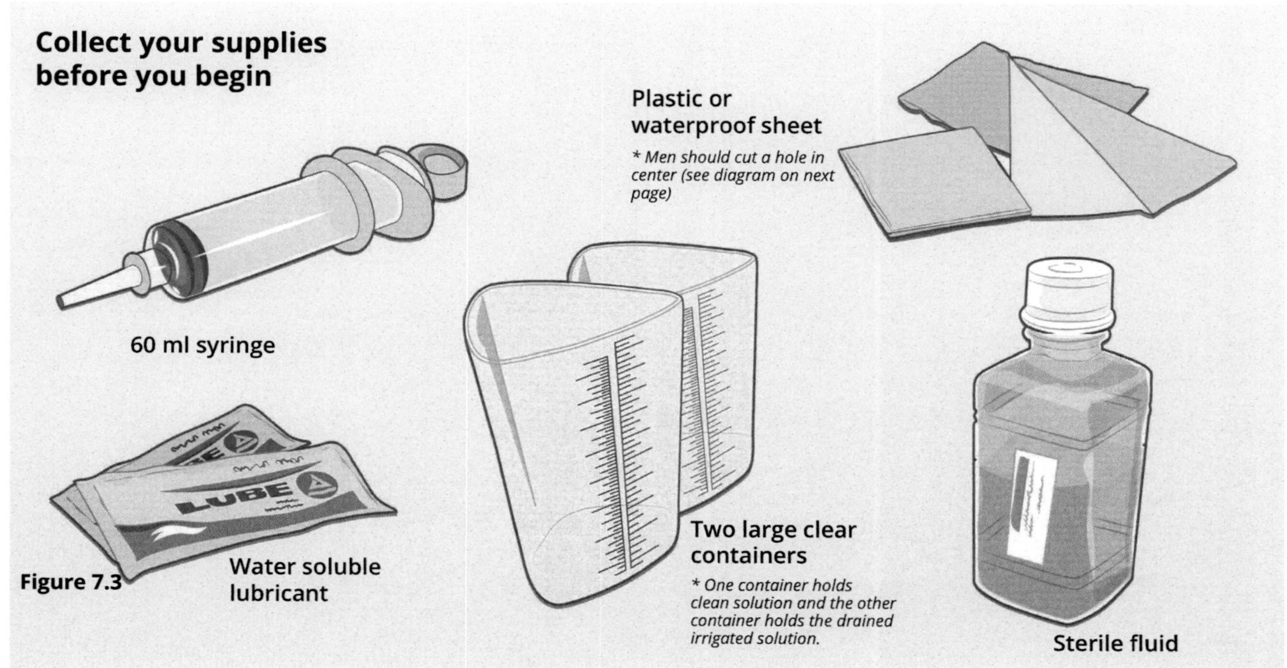

Figure 7.3

your catheter and cause urine to leak or your bladder to spasm. If you see any blood in your urine, drink more fluids until your urine clears. Call your doctor immediately if your urine stops draining for more than two hours.

You may need to flush your catheter. Irrigating your bladder is a way to wash out your bladder. Flushing sterile fluid into your bladder helps to clear a blockage and wash out blood clots.

Steps for Irrigating Your Bladder

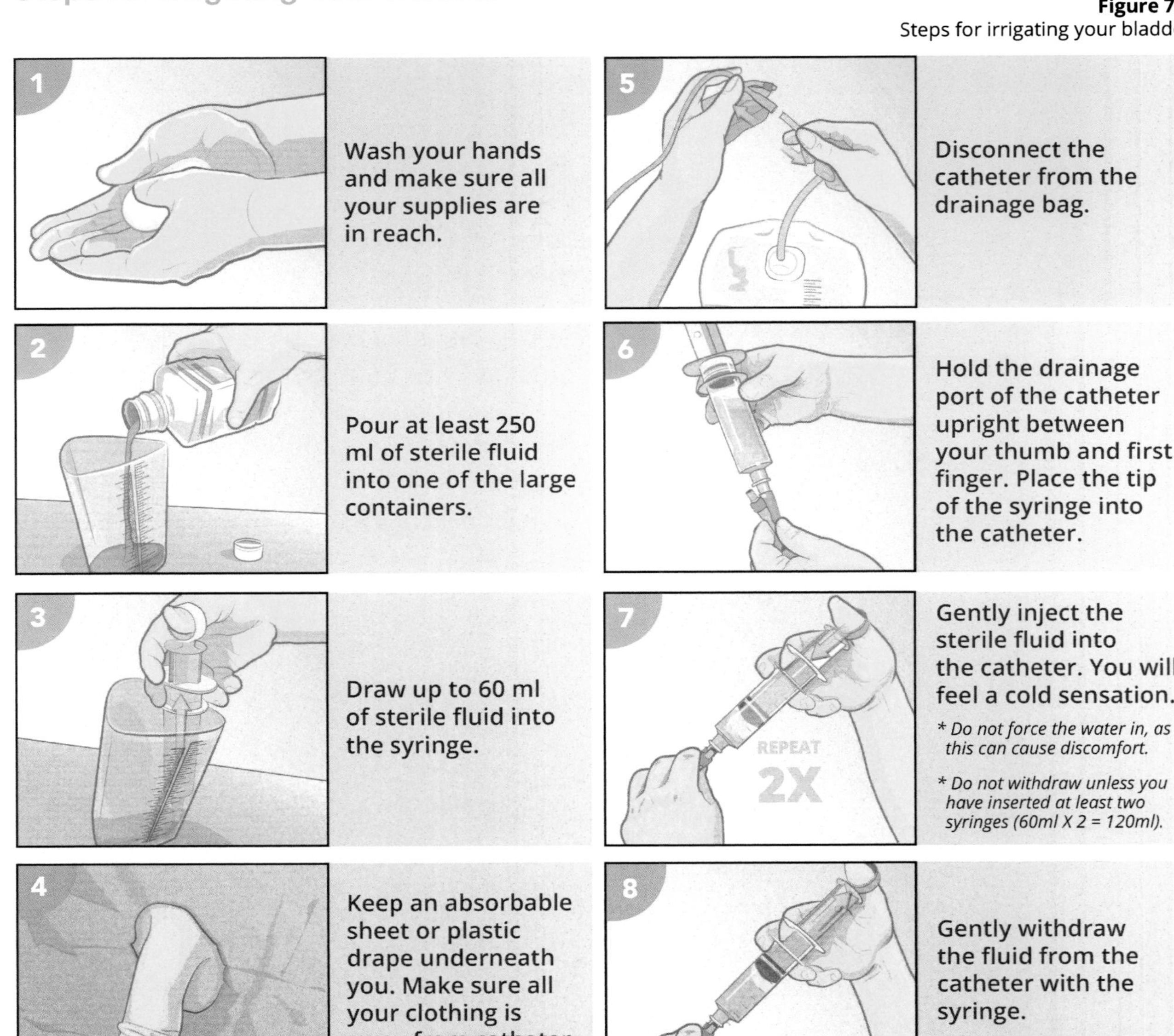

Figure 7.4
Steps for irrigating your bladder

Call your doctor immediately if you experience:

- Any sign of infection: fever of 101.5° F or higher.
- Excessive bleeding in or around the catheter.
- No urine draining from the catheter, even though you have been drinking plenty of fluids.
- A lot of urine leaking around the catheter, despite trying the measures explained above.
- Urine that is cloudy or has a thick consistency.

How to Describe Any Bleeding to Your Physician

Clear
Light Tinge with No Blood Clots
Slightly Darker
Thick with Small Blood Clots
Fresh Blood Clots
WATER
TOMATO KETCHUP
Water
Fruit Punch
Ketchup

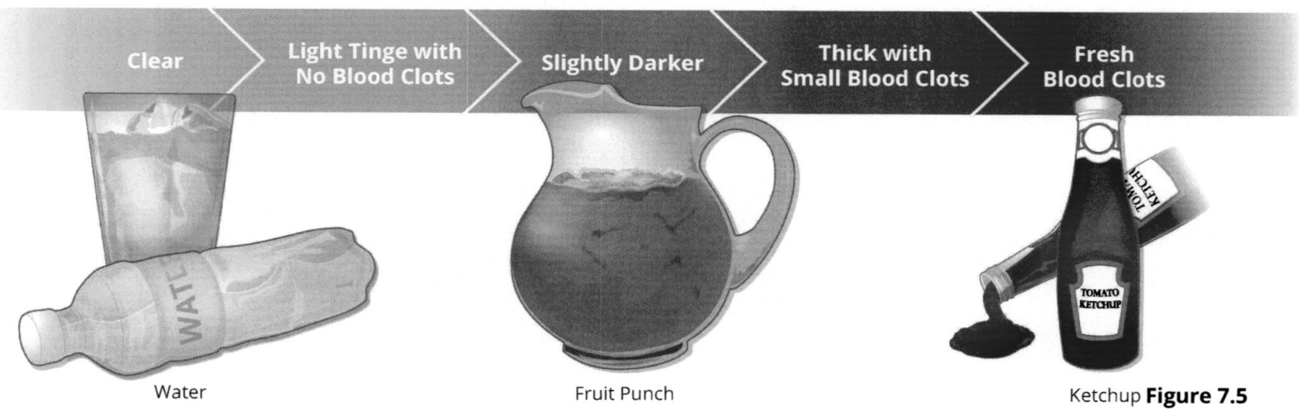

Figure 7.5

Chapter 8

What Did the Pathology Show?

HOW DO I UNDERSTAND MY PATHOLOGY?

Your doctor sends the abnormal cells or tumor tissue obtained during your trans-urethral surgery to a pathology laboratory for further testing and examination under a microscope. The pathology report gives your doctor valuable information about your tumor, which helps determine the best treatment for your specific case. The pathology report also tells your doctor more about your cancer's shape (morphology) and cell type (histology).

Terms You Should Know

Pathology
This branch of medical science primarily involves the examination of tissues, organs and bodily fluids to study and diagnose disease.

Tumor
Any abnormal growth of cells, whether benign or malignant.

Low Grade Tumor
Low grade tumors are tumors that cannot invade neighboring tissues or spread to other parts of the body. Generally cells often resemble the original tissue and grow slowly. These are not cancer.

Malignant Tumor
Malignant tumors are cancer. They can invade neighboring tissues and spread to other parts of the body. Cells usually grow out of control.

Metastasis
When cancer (a malignant tumor) spreads to distant areas of the body, far from the cancer's original site. A tumor that has spread and begins to grow in another site is called a metastatic tumor.

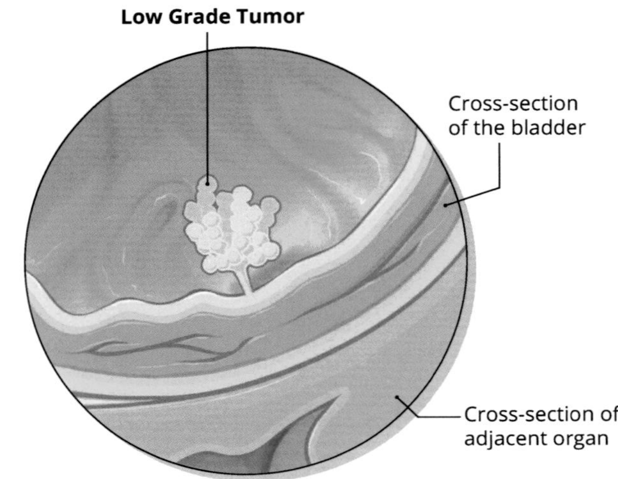

Figure 8.1 a
Illustrated cross-section of the bladder with a low-grade tumor

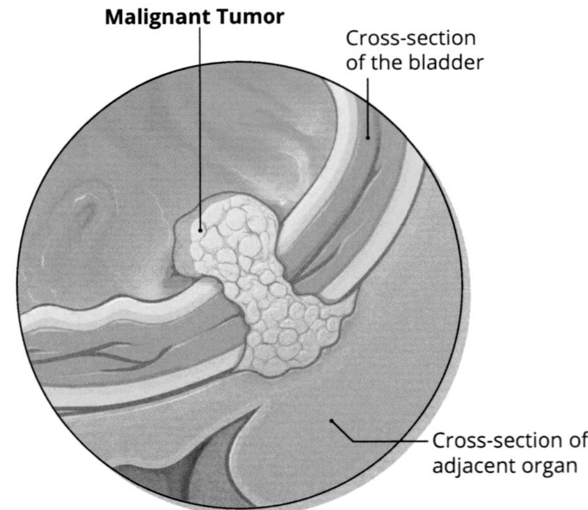

Figure 8.1 b
Illustrated cross-section of the bladder with a malignant tumor

Tumor Morphology (Shape)

The shape of your cancer can tell your doctor how serious your cancer is and help determine the best way to remove it. Both papillary and flat tumors can be noninvasive (*in situ*) or invasive (grows into and/or through the other bladder layers).

Flat Tumors

These superficial, flat, spreading tumors are also called sessile tumors. These tumors are often more difficult to treat.

Papillary Tumors

These tumors have long, finger-like projections that stretch out from the bladder wall towards your bladder's interior.

Histological Types

Histology is the study of the microscopic structure of cells. The most common type of cancer cells in the bladder is the transitional cell carcinoma (approximately 90%). Other histological types of cancer cells include: squamous cell carcinoma, adenocarcinoma, and small cell carcinoma (which include neuroendocrine, micropapillary and mixed-pattern subtypes) and sarcoma.

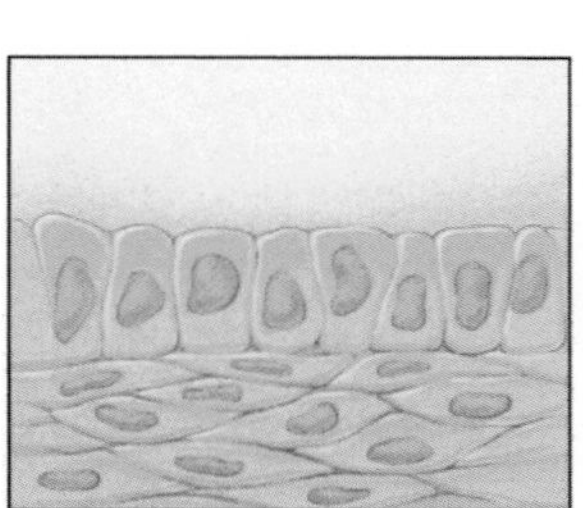

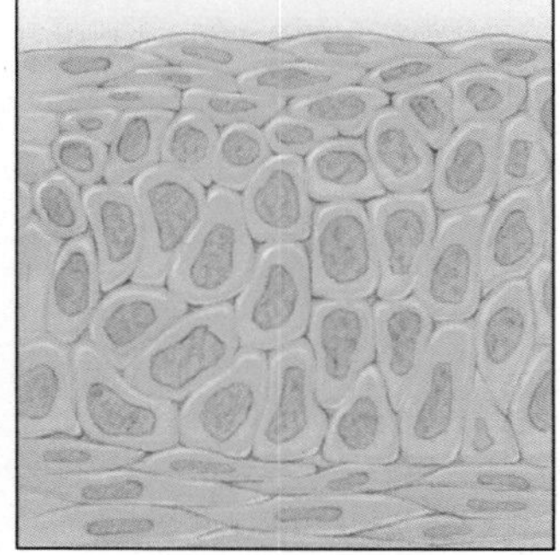

Figure 8.2
Side by side comparison of normal cells versus cancer cells as viewed under a microscope

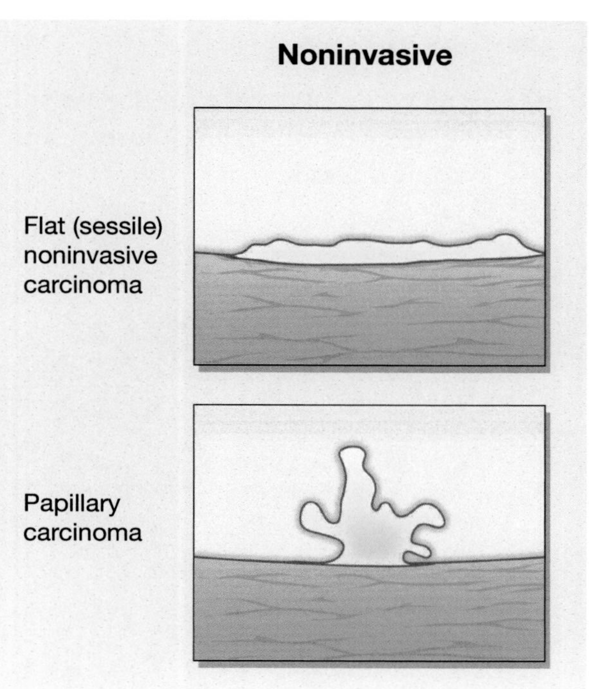

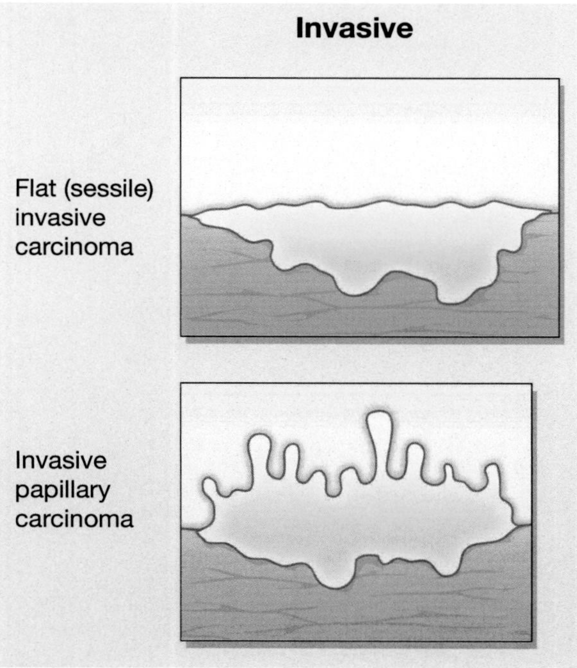

Figure 8.3
Invasive and noninvasive tumor morphology

Stages of Cancer

Understanding the stage of your disease will help you understand the natural history and course of your disease.

T - Describes the tumor shape and depth
N - Whether any lymph nodes have cancer
M - Metastasis

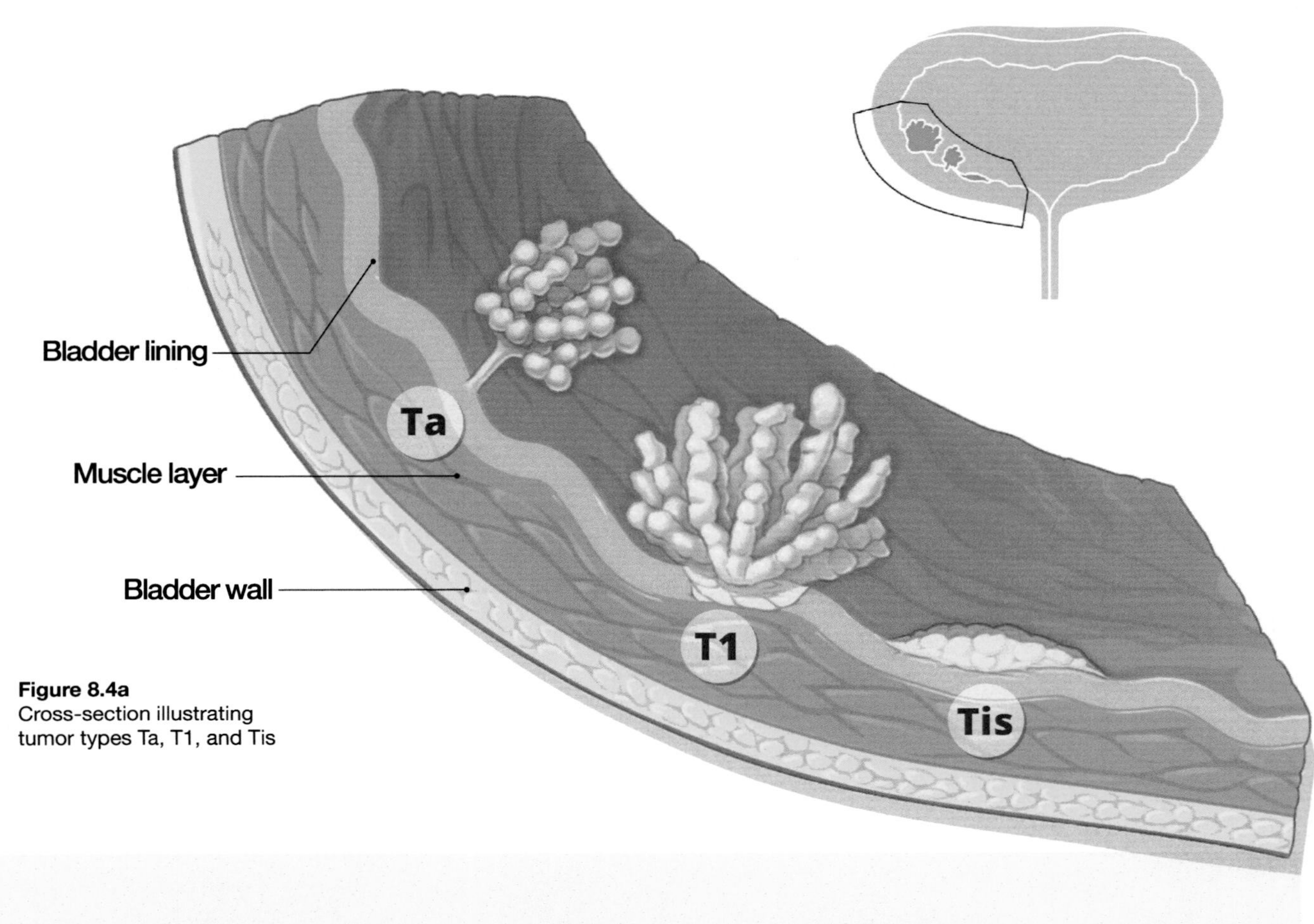

Figure 8.4a
Cross-section illustrating tumor types Ta, T1, and Tis

	Ta	T1	Tis
Pathological Classification	**Noninvasive papillary carcinoma**	**Tumor invades bladder lining**	**Carcinoma *in situ* (i.e. flat tumor)**
Translation	The bladder cancer is papillary shaped and limited to the innermost layer of the bladder.	The tumor has extended into the second layer of the bladder, but has not reached the muscle layer.	The bladder cancer is flat and spreading, but is limited to the innermost layer of the bladder.

Figure 8.4b
Cross-section illustrating tumor types T2, T3, and T4

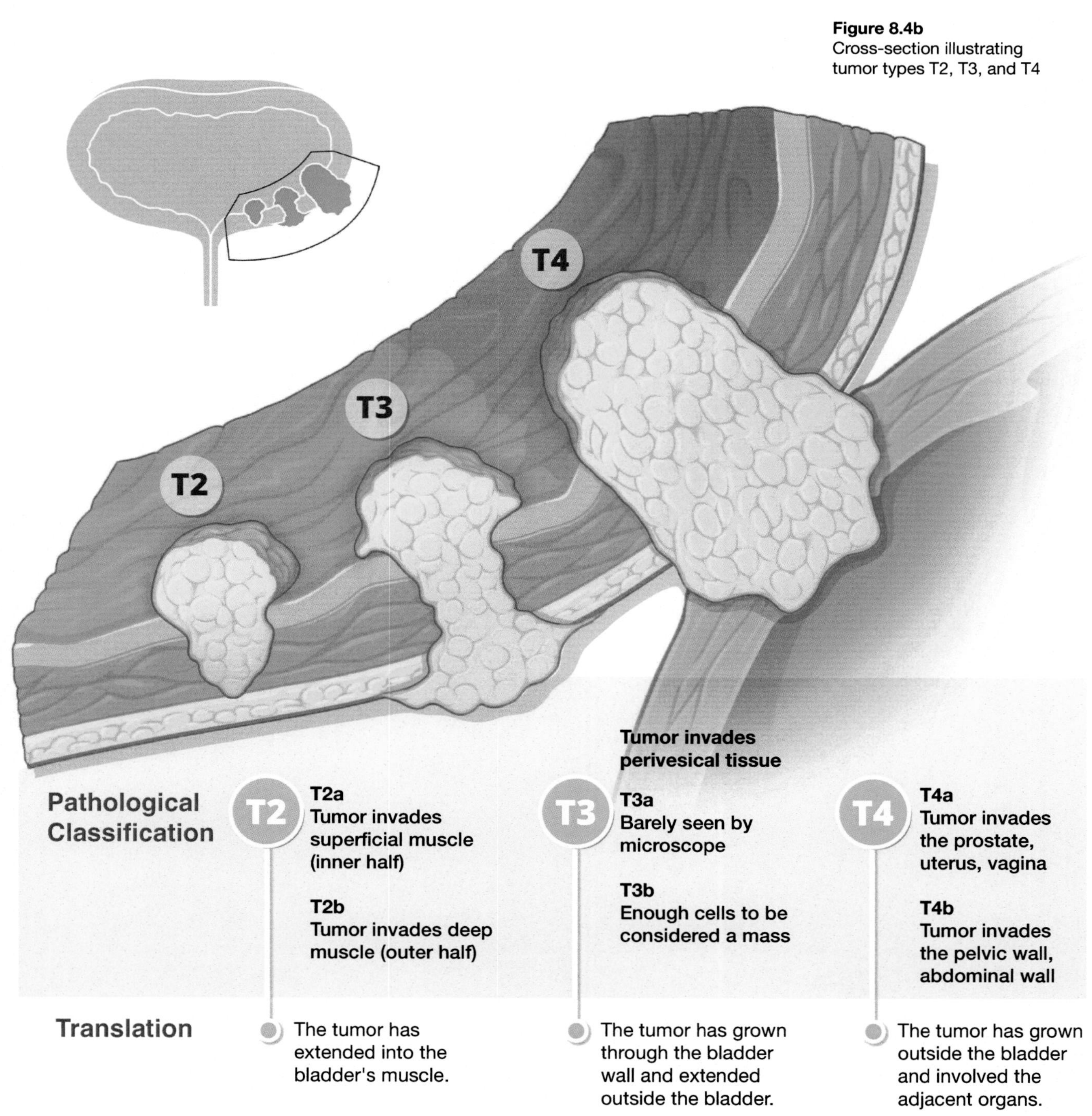

Lymph Nodes

Lymph nodes are small organs found throughout the body that enlarge when infected or when invaded by cancer cells.

The nodes surrounding the bladder area are removed during the cystectomy to see if any cancer cells are found in them. If so, this indicates that the cancer has begun to spread.

Pathological Classification	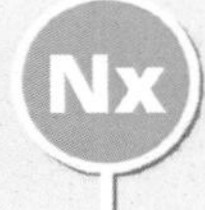 **Nx** **Lymph nodes were not examined**	 **N0** **No regional lymph node metastasis**	 **N1** **Metastasis in a single lymph node in the true pelvis** **(hypogastric, obturator, external iliac or presacral)**
Translation	Lymph nodes were not examined	The examined lymph nodes are cancer-free	Cancer cells were found in a single lymph node near your bladder

Pathological Classification	 **N2** **Metastasis in multiple lymph nodes in the true pelvis** **(hypogastric, obturator, external iliac or presacral)**	**N3** **Metastasis in common iliac lymph nodes**
Translation	Cancer cells were found in more than one lymph node near your bladder	Cancer cells were found in lymph nodes distant from the bladder.

Figure 8.5
The different stages of cancer spread to the lymph nodes.

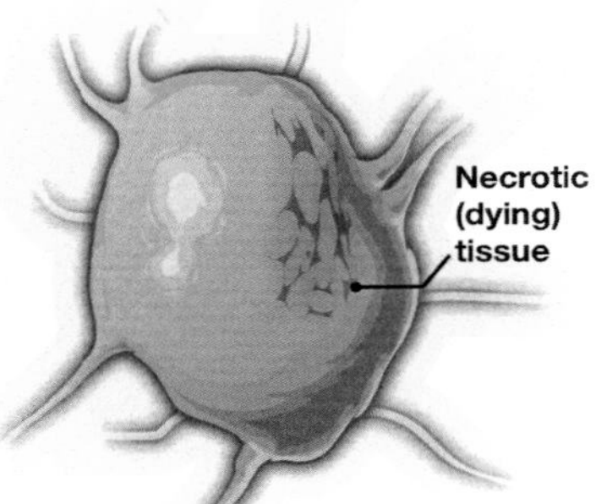

Figure 8.6
Comparison of normal and cancerous lymph nodes

Metastasis

Metastasis means that cells from the bladder cancer have spread to other organs. Other common sites that may be affected include lung, bone and lymph nodes.

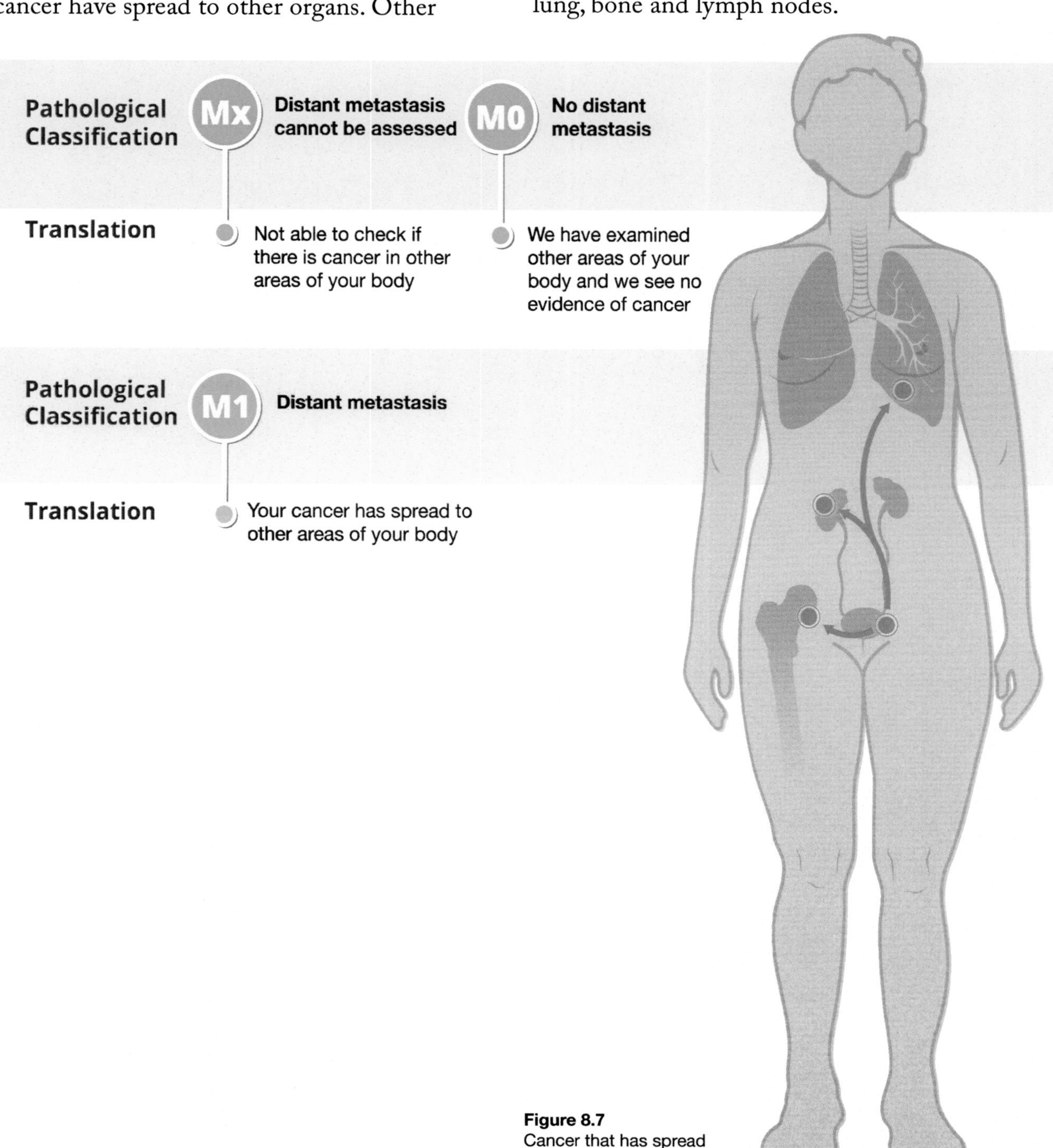

Figure 8.7
Cancer that has spread to other organs

Risk stratification is used by your surgeon to evaluate the complexity of your disease. You may discuss your pathology and this chart with your surgeon.

American Urologic Association Risk Stratification for Non-Muscle-Invasive Bladder Cancer

Low Risk	Intermediate Risk	High Risk
Low-grade solitary Ta ≤3cm	Recurrence within 1 year, low-grade Ta	High-grade T1
Papillary urothelial neoplasm of low malignant potential	Solitary Ta > 3cm	Recurrent Ta high-grade
	Low-grade Ta, multifocal	High-grade Ta, >3 cm or multifocal
	High-grade Ta, ≤3cm	Carcinoma *in situ*
	Low-grade T1	BCG failure in high-grade
		Variant histology
		Lymphovascular invasion
		High-grade in prostatic urethra

Chapter 9

Intravesical Treatment: Inserting Medication into the Bladder

INTRAVESICAL THERAPY

After your tumor is removed by your surgeon, your doctor will determine if you should have additional medical treatment using drugs to fight your cancer. If so, you will have to wait for the wound from the tumor removal to heal and form a scar inside your bladder, it usually takes three to six weeks.

You should not have intravesical chemotherapy if your TURBT may have perforated your bladder, or resulted in an extensive surgery, or tumor resection or you have gross hematuria (visible blood in urine).

With Intravesical therapy (IVT), doctors place a liquid medication directly into the bladder through a catheter, rather than giving it by mouth or injecting into the blood. The main advantage of this method is that the drug can directly affect the cells within the bladder without circulating through your body and causing major side effects. The main side effects of intravesical therapy are irritation and a burning feeling in the bladder.

Which Drugs Will I Have?

Your doctor will choose the drugs best for you based on your individual diagnosis. Your IVT may use chemotherapy drugs such as mitomycin C, gemcitabine, valrubicin, and BCG. Most commonly, mitomycin C is used for IVT right after surgery as a single dose. Some research suggests that heating the inside of the bladder improves the effectiveness of mitomycin C.

How is IVT given?
First, a catheter (thin tube) is inserted through your urethra into your bladder. Then, the liquid medication is put into the catheter and flows into your bladder. The medication needs to stay in your bladder for two hours.

Intravesical Immunotherapy

Immunotherapy uses drugs designed to provoke your own immune system to attack the cancer cells. Immunotherapy drugs may also be placed directly in your bladder with IVT.

One type of immunotherapy drug, Bacillus Calmentte-Guerin (BCG) is a weakened form of the bacteria that causes tuberculosis. Placing the BCG directly into your bladder triggers your immune system to attack the cancer cells in your bladder and may stop the future growth of cancer cells, too.

You may be treated once a week for six weeks. After the first six weeks you may need treatments (maintenance) only once a month for between one to three years. Follow up with imaging scans, cystoscopy and cytology is important.

What are the side effects of BCG?
Your may experience painful, frequent, or urgent urination for three to five days after treatment. Other side effects may include:

- Nausea (upset stomach), occasional vomiting
- Flu-like symptoms (fever, chills), which may occur between four and eight hours after receiving BCG
- Loss of appetite
- Difficulty urinating or blood in your urine

- Fever (above 100.4° F or 38°C)
- Joint pain
- Cough
- Skin rash

What are rare, but possible side effects of BCG?

Side effects from an allergic reaction or blood infection (sepsis) can occur within a week of BCG treatments. These reactions are rare, but when they do occur, it is serious. You may need to be treated in the hospital.

Allergic reaction occurs when your body's immune system overreacts to a foreign substance.
Sepsis is a serious infection that has spread throughout your body.

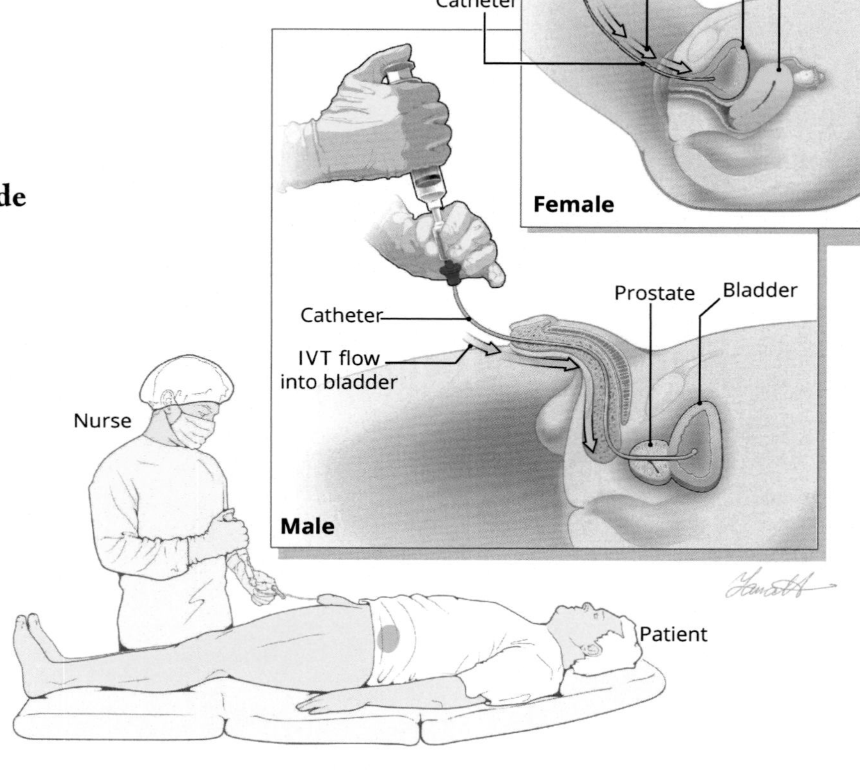

Figure 9.1
IVT administration in male and female

Call your doctor immediately if you experience any signs of an allergic reaction:

- Itching
- Hives
- Swelling of your face or hands
- Swelling or tingling in your mouth or throat
- Tightness in your chest

Get medical attention immediately if you have:

- Fever of 103° F (39°C) for more than 24 hours, or a fever with chills
- Severe shivering
- Dizziness or feeling light-headed
- Confusion
- Shortness of breath
- Weakness

The IVT Procedure

It is important to follow the treatment instructions carefully, for two main reasons:

1. **Safety**
Following the instructions will help keep others from getting sick. Direct contact with the medication or drugs in your urine or other body fluids (by using the same toilet you use or if you have sex without a condom) can sicken others.

2. **Better response**
IVT may not work effectively if the instructions are not followed.

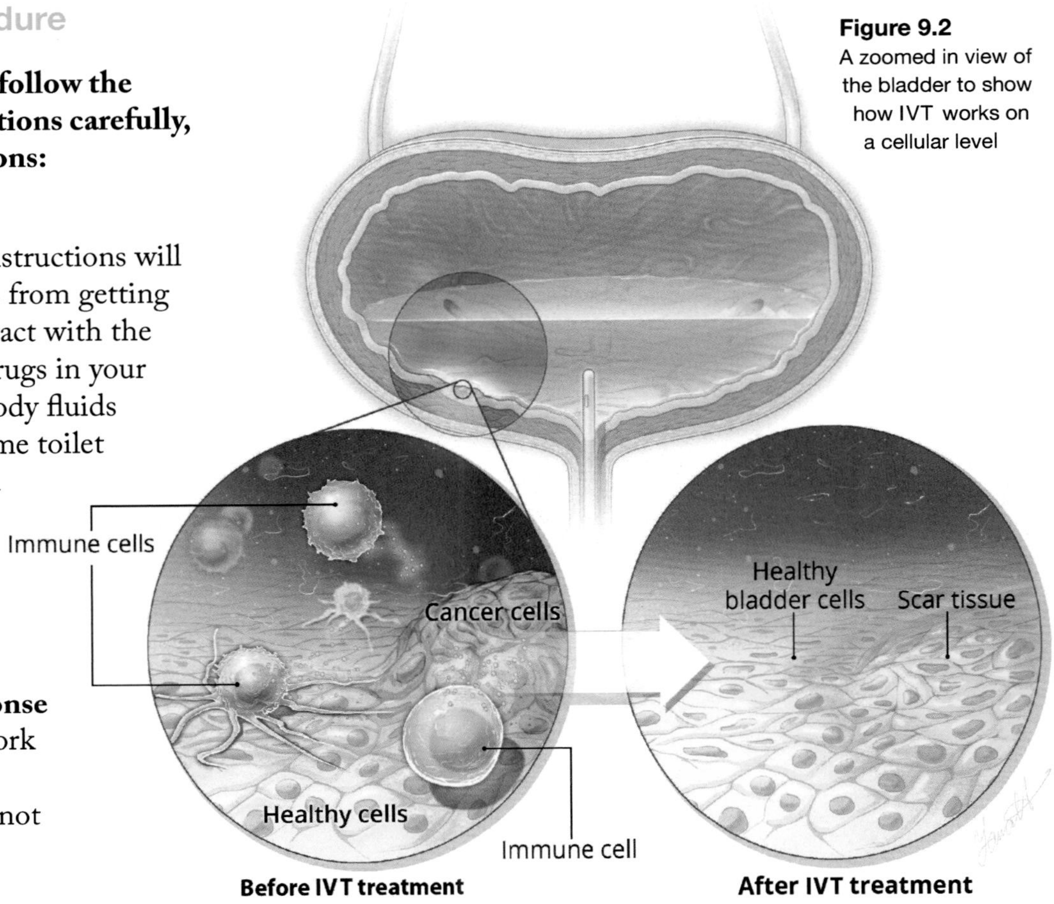

Figure 9.2
A zoomed in view of the bladder to show how IVT works on a cellular level

Before treatment begins, tell your doctor if:

- You are taking any medications, vitamins, herbs or diet supplements
- You have any allergies
- You received the smallpox vaccine recently
- You have ever had a positive test for tuberculosis (TB)
- You have a fever, infection, severe burn or immune disorder
- You are pregnant or breastfeeding

You should not undergo IVT treatment if:

- There is any difficulty inserting a catheter
- You have blood (visible to the naked eye) in your urine
- You have a urinary tract infection (UTI)
- You had a bladder biopsy or surgery (such as TURBT) within the past seven to 14 days

Preparing for Treatment

Starting four hours before your treatment:

- Do not drink any liquids. If you drink liquids, there may not be enough room in your bladder for the drugs.
- Do not empty your bladder (pee).

Once treatment has begun, the drugs must stay in your bladder for up to two hours.

- If you are able to hold it in for the full two hours, you may go home to complete the rest of the treatment.
- If you are not able to hold it in, you will remain in the clinic for two hours with the catheter in place. A clamp will be placed on the catheter to hold the drugs in your bladder.

You may be asked to change positions so that the medication washes over all areas of your bladder.

Instruction After Each Treatment

Two hours after treatment

Whether you go home or stay in the clinic, do not drink any liquids for two hours. After two hours have passed, drink plenty of liquids to flush out the medication.

Six hours after treatment:

- You may take acetaminophen (Tylenol) for any fever or pain or diphenhydramine (Benadryl) for itching if needed.
- To avoid splashing urine, both men and women should sit down to urinate. Splashed urine exposes other people to the drugs in your urine which could make them ill.

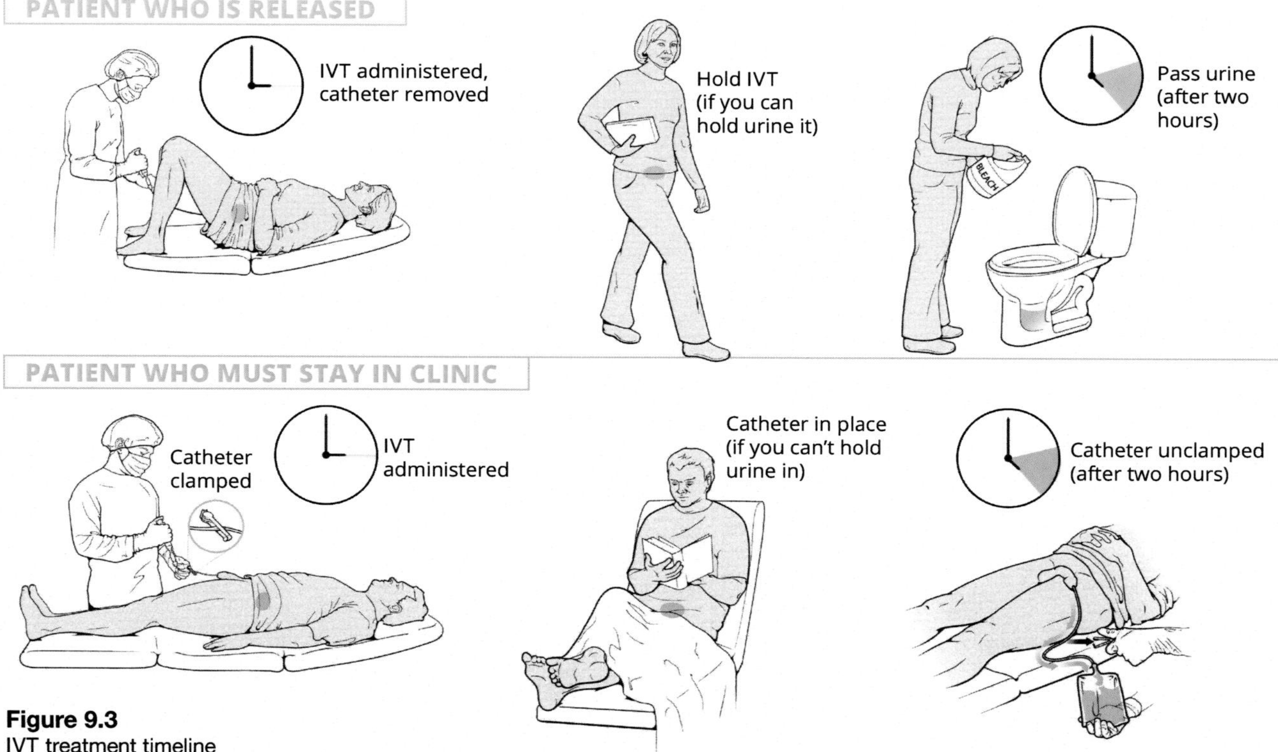

Figure 9.3
IVT treatment timeline

- After you urinate, pour two cups of full-strength bleach (not diluted) into the toilet, wait 15 minutes and then close the lid and flush. This will help protect other people from getting sick from any drugs in your urine.
- Wash your genitals after you urinate. This will help protect your skin from getting irritated by the drugs in your urine.

For 48 hours after treatment
Do not masturbate or have any type of sex with another person. Masturbating can cause the drugs to get on your hands or genitals. Having sex with another person could cause that person to become ill from being exposed to the drugs from your body.

For six weeks after treatment
Always use a condom during sex to protect your partner from the live IVT drugs. Avoid pregnancy. We do not know how IVT affects sperm, eggs, embryos, or fetuses.

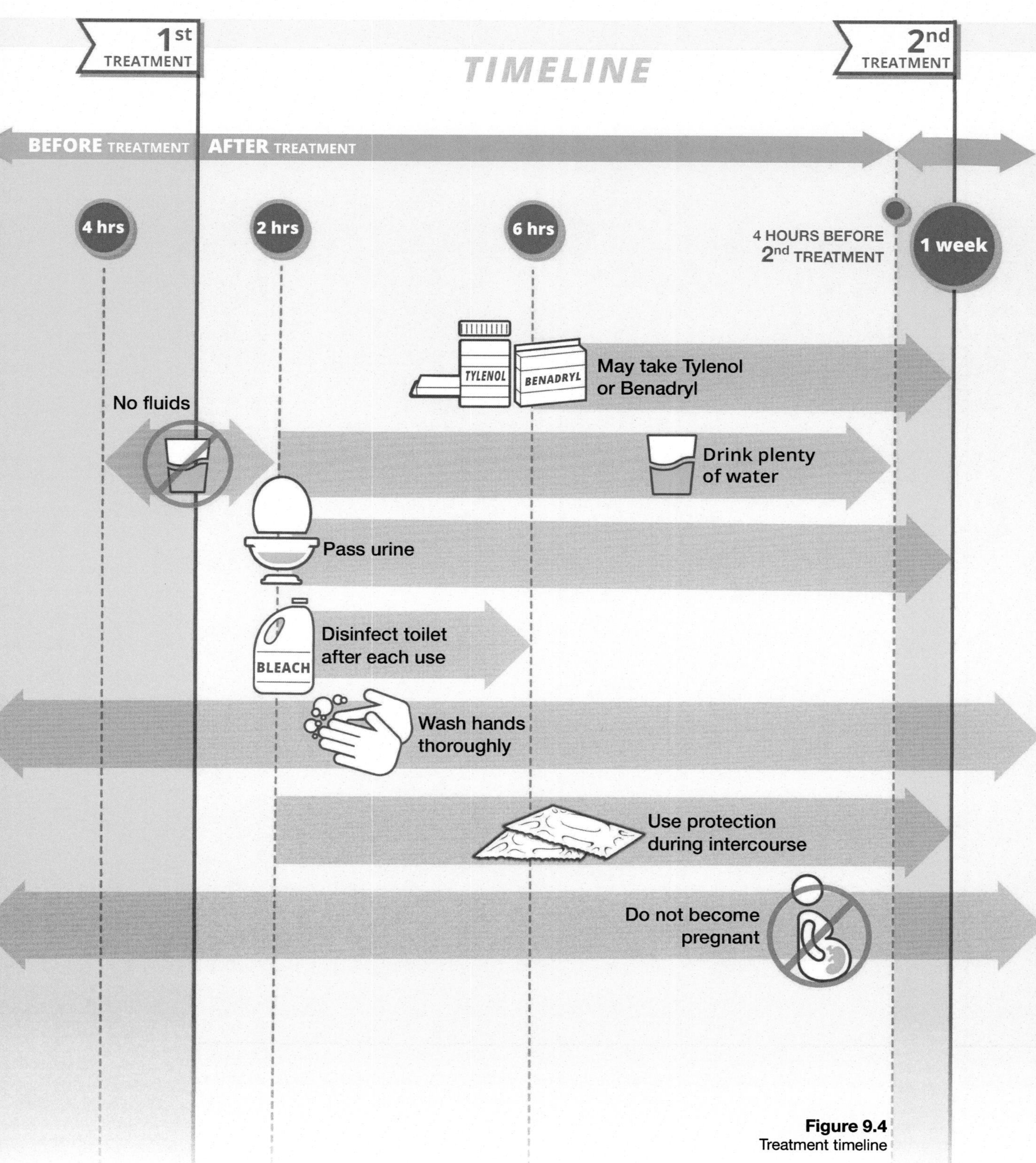

Figure 9.4
Treatment timeline

FREQUENTLY ASKED QUESTIONS:

Q: Will a tuberculosis test (PPD) be positive after BCG treatment?

A: Yes

Q: Can I receive BCG treatment if I test positive for tuberculosis (TB)?

A: Yes

Q: Can I be around a pregnant woman after I receive BCG treatment?

A: Yes

Q: Can I get tuberculosis (TB) if I forget to clean the toilet while being treated with BCG?

A: Yes. It is rare, but it can still occur.

Q: Should I worry if I have blood in my urine after treatment?

A: No. (But call your doctor if you have a lot of blood and your urine has a ketchup-color and consistency. If blood is persistent it may delay the next treatment.)

Q: Can I have BCG treatment if I take medicines that weaken the immune system (for example, prednisone)?

A: No. Tell your doctor about all your medications before treatment.

Chapter 10

Preparing For Surgery

YOUR PRE-OPERATIVE VISIT

You and your physician team have decided that surgery is needed to treat your cancer. The clock starts now. We recommend using the following flow chart and writing all key dates in your calendar. This will help you prepare for surgery in a safe and thorough manner.

This visit is a special doctor's appointment that is **scheduled within a month before your surgery** to see how prepared you and your body are for the stress and postsurgical effects. You will meet with different members of your team and have some tests done to see if, for any reason, you will be at risk during or after the surgery.

What You Should Know

- If you are having cystoscopy/TURBT, you may go home the same day or spend the night (or two nights, which is rare) in the hospital.
    - Patients who have this surgery may be put to sleep with anesthesia (medications that keep you unconscious during the operation).
    - Depending on how extensive your surgery is, you may go home that day, spend the night in the hospital, or spend several days in the hospital to recover.
- If you are having a cystectomy, you will be hospitalized for several days following your surgery.

On the Day of Your Visit

A health provider will make some basic assessments, such as your height, weight temperature, blood pressure and heart rate.

Afterward either a physician, physician's assistant, or nurse practitioner will take your full medical history and conduct a physical examination. They will ask you about any allergies, medical issues or surgeries you may have had in the past as well as any medications you currently take. Bring a list of your medications.

The medical team will tell you which medications to **stop or change** before the surgery. Tell your doctor about any health changes before surgery.

Figure 10.1
Your preoperative timeline, detailed on pages 55-57

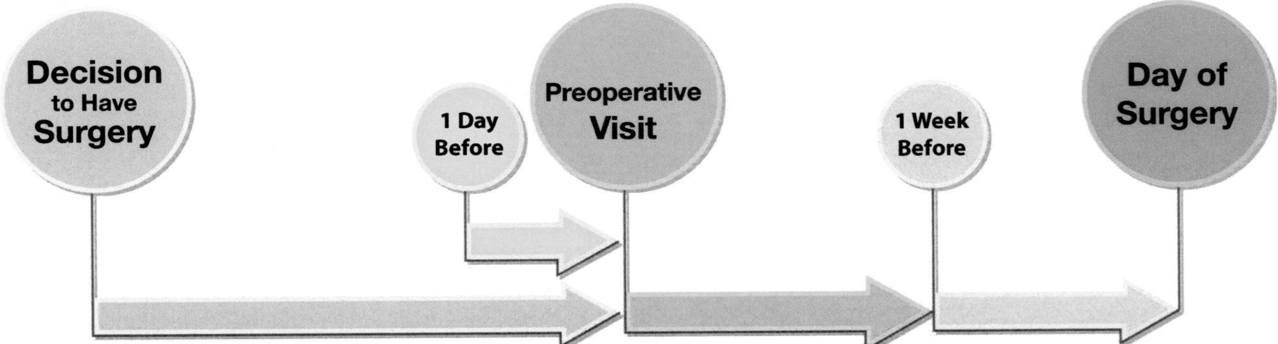

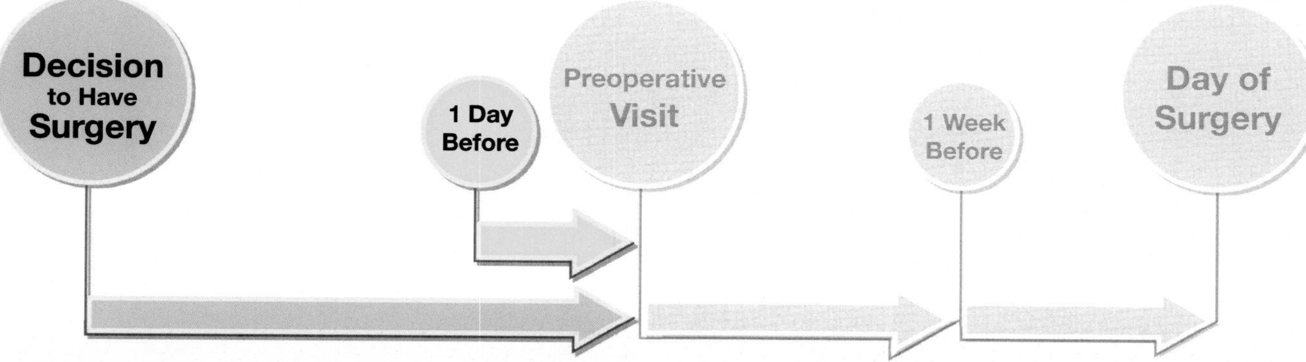

Decision Day → Preoperative Visit

Between the decision day and the day of the preop appointment you should:

- Learn and understand the risks and benefits of your procedure.
- Consider your overall health and major medical issues, with special attention to diabetes and heart and lung problems.
- Make sure your surgical team has your updated heart and lungs (cardiopulmonary) status. Get your records; contact your heart and lung specialists.
- Make sure your team has a record of medications you are taking and any allergies you have.
- Have your nutritional status evaluated if advised.
- Ask to connect with patients who have undergone similar surgery by your surgeon.
- Stop smoking.
- Keep moving. Be as active as your health allows.
- Prepare a Living Will and Health Care Proxy. Discuss your wishes with your family.
- Look for an advocacy (support) group and attend a meeting.
- Discuss your surgery with your family or friends so they can take time off or travel with you.
- Use incentive spirometer or practice deep breathing exercises.

1 Day Before → Preoperative Visit

One day before your preop appointment, you should:

- Make sure all other consultants or physicians (e.g., pulmonologist, cardiologist) have sent their recommendations.
- Discuss any changes or events that took place since your decision to have surgery.
- If you have a pacemaker, bring the card which describes its details.
- Bring copies of your Living Will and Health Care Proxy.
- Bring a family member or a friend with you.
- Write down any questions to ask.

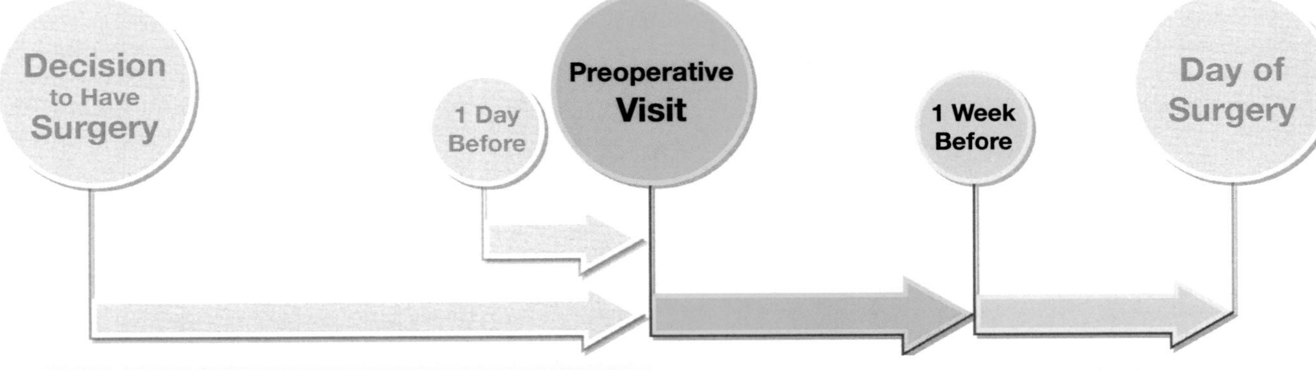

Preoperative Visit

At your preop visit, your health provider will:

- Check your vital signs, take your medical history, and perform a thorough physical exam.
- Check all blood tests, imaging reports, and additional tests (CT, lung function, echocardiogram, etc.)
- Review the recommendations from your other doctors.
- Discuss all your current medications and your allergies and give you instructions if you need to stop any medications before surgery.
- Review the surgery and discuss the risks.
- Tell you how to prepare for day of surgery and what to expect.
- Provide you with a dietary plan.
- Ask if you will be able to care for yourself after surgery.

1 Week Before → Day of Surgery

The week before your surgery you should:

- Stop taking blood-thinning medications (e.g., aspirin, Plavix, Coumadin, Eliquis, Lovenox) if your surgeon and the doctor who prescribed them are *in agreement* about stopping these important medications.
- Stop taking anti inflammatory pain medications, generally three to five days before surgery.
- Prepare updated list of your medications, dosages and how often you take them, *especially if it has changed* since you saw your surgeons.
- Confirm which medications you should still take on the day of surgery.
- Tell your anesthesiologist if you have had problems with anesthesia before.
- Tell your surgeon immediately if you get a cold, an infection, or any other health change.
- Make copies of your Advanced Directive and Health Care Proxy and bring them with you.
- Arrange for someone to drive you home after your surgery. If you have same-day (outpatient) surgery, you will not be allowed to drive.
- Follow instructions about when to have your last solid meal and liquids.

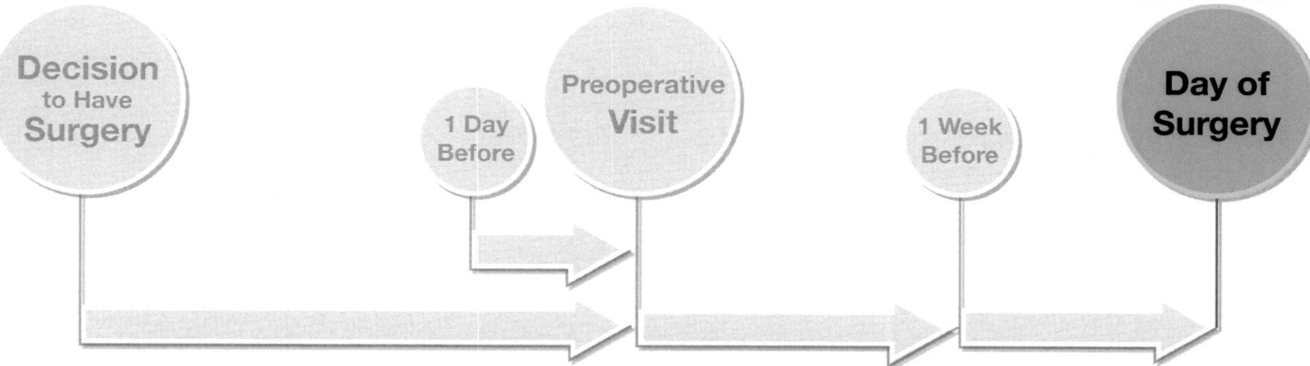

Day of Surgery

The day of your surgery you should:

- Take appropriate medications as instructed.
- Be prepared to talk about any changes in your health or medications.
- Remove any nail polish, piercings, or jewelry.
- Bring your CPAP machine for sleep apnea if you use one and are staying in the hospital.
- Bring copies of your Advanced Directive, Health Care Proxy, an updated list of medications, and a list of allergies.
- Pack your bag with personal items, such as toiletries, eye glasses and reading materials.
- DO NOT bring any valuables, including credit cards, jewelry, or money to the hospital.
- Bathe the morning of your procedure or the night before.
- DO NOT apply body lotions, deodorant or powder after taking your shower.
- DO NOT shave anywhere near your operation site. Brush your teeth, swish, spit. Remove contact lenses. You may bring a storage lens case or an extra pair of eyeglasses.
- If appropriate, bring your crutches or walker with you, labeled with your contact information.
- Wear loose-fitting clothing, preferably a button-down shirt
- Provide emergency contact information (name and phone number). Let your team know if your emergency contact will be with you or available remotely.

Medication Restrictions*

- **7 days prior to surgery**
  Stop taking aspirin, clopidogrel, Plavix, herbal supplements and vitamins.
- **5 days prior to surgery**
  Stop taking warfarin (Coumadin).
- **3 days prior to surgery**
  Stop taking NSAIDs, such as ibuprofen and naproxen sodium (Advil, Motrin, and Aleve).
- **2 days prior to surgery**
  Stop taking daltparin (Fragmin), fondaparinux, Arixtra.
- **1 day prior to surgery**
  Stop taking enoxaparin.
- **Day of your surgery**
  Take only the medications your doctor says are okay, with small amounts of water.
  **As advised by your physician*

Diet

- **Day before surgery**
  Follow a clear liquid diet, drinking only liquids that you can see through (Gatorade, ginger ale or water).
- **After midnight, the night before your surgery**
  Do not eat or drink anything except the medicine your doctor approved, with only a little bit of water. If you are having a cystectomy, your surgeons may want your bowels to be clear during the operation. Your physician may allow you to drink and eat up to two hours before surgery if you are following the the ERAS pathway (see Chapter 13).

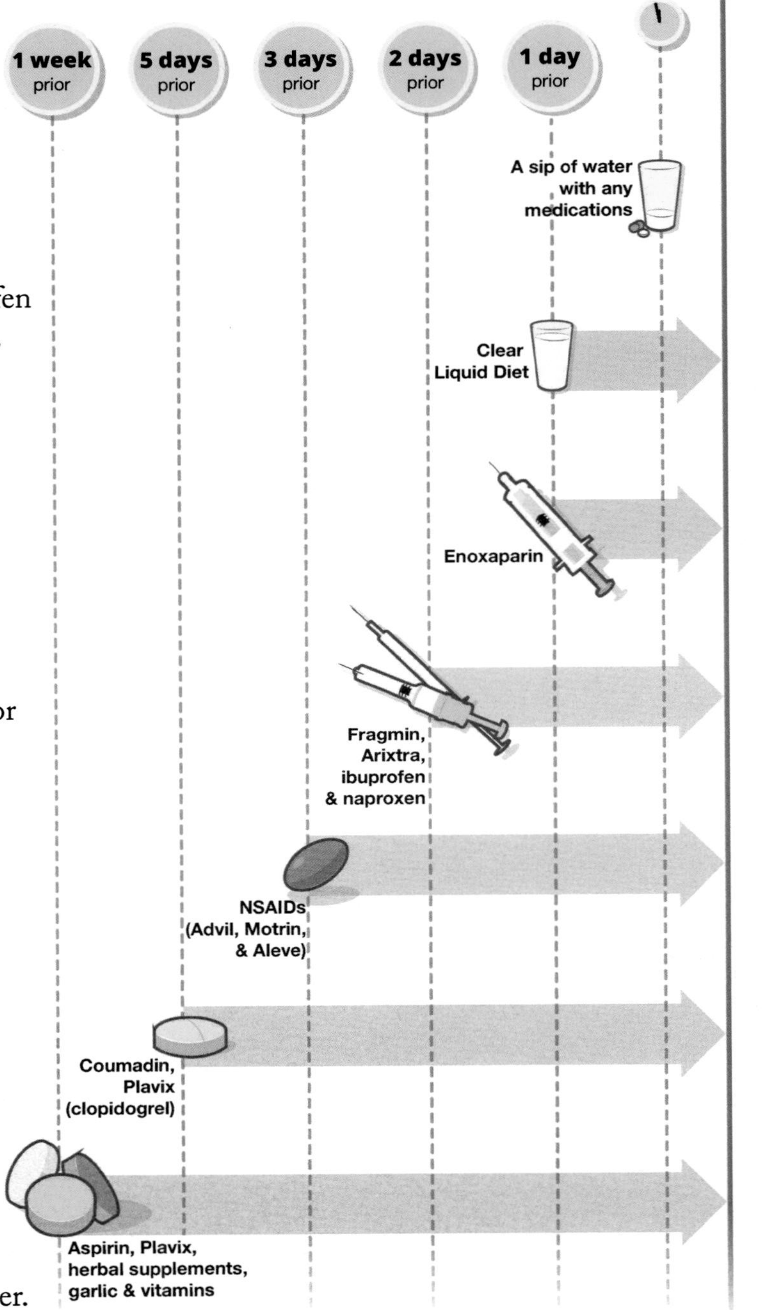

Figure 10.2
Preoperative timeline of restrictions of commonly used medications

On Your Pre-Op Day

Your healthcare provider team will conduct any tests your doctor orders to identify any risks you may face, and help your medical team prepare for your specific surgery. Some common tests include:

Blood Tests

Blood tests determine your blood type and cell count, and indicate whether you may be at risk for infection or whether you might need a transfusion.

Chest X-ray

To gauge your lung function, you might be given an incentive **spirometer,** a device that measures your lung volume and helps you perform breathing exercises. This exercises expand your lungs and **helps prevent pneumonia** as you recover after your surgery.

Echocardiogram Electrocardiogram and/or Stress Test

An echocardiogram, electrocardiogram (EKG), and/or stress tests will check your heart's performance and help determine whether it can handle the added stress of surgery.

Imaging

Imaging, such as CT scans and/or MRIs look at your other organs.

How Can I Improve My Outcome?

- Stop smoking.
- Take medications as directed.
- Be as active as you can safely be. Daily physical activity is best, if your doctor allows it.
- Use incentive spirometer.

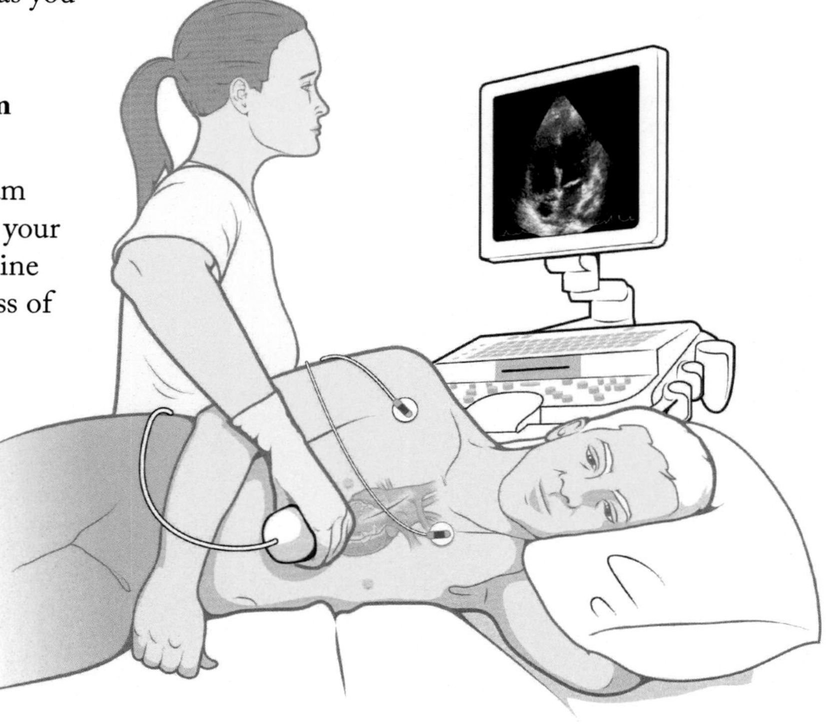

Figure 10.3
Medical professional performing a cardiac echocardiogram

Spirometer Breathing Exercises

1. Stand or sit up straight.
2. Hold the spirometer upright.
3. **Exhale**, then close your lips tightly around the mouthpiece.
4. **Inhale**, as if sipping liquid through a straw, to lift the three balls to the top of the device.

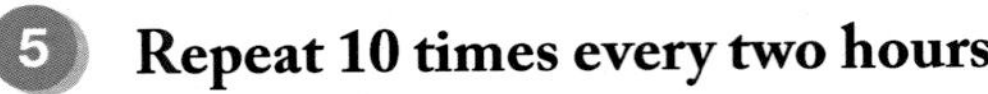

5. **Repeat 10 times every two hours.**

Your Goal: Work up to lifting all three balls and holding them up for 10 seconds. Holding one ball up for 10 seconds is better than getting two balls up for one second. **Hold the balls up by taking slow, deep breaths.**

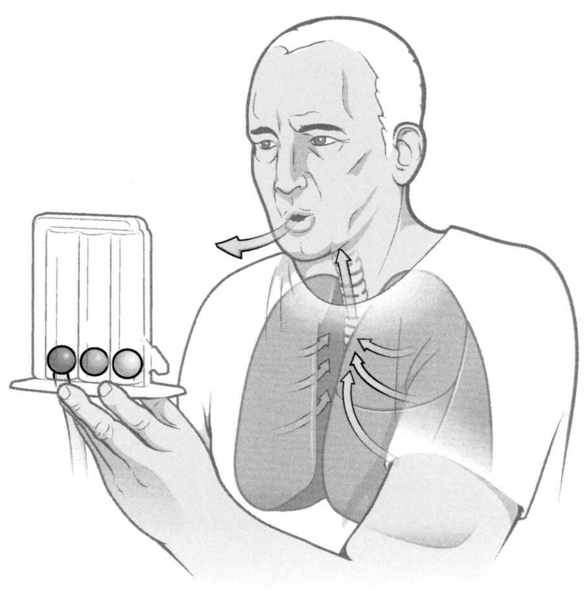

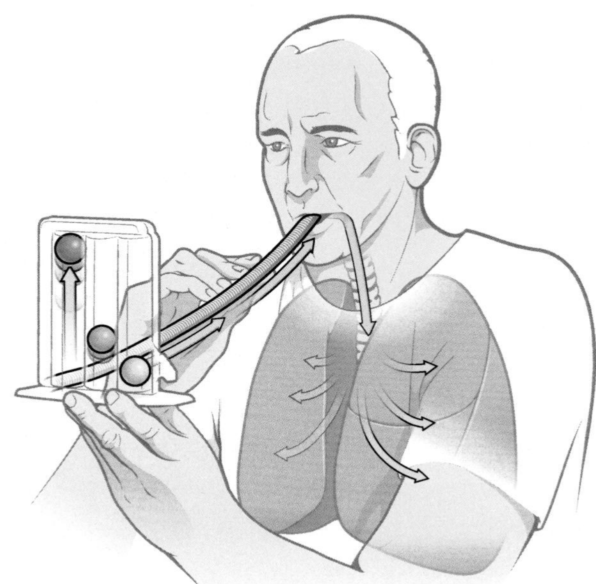

Figure 10.4
Patient performing the breathing exercise using a spirometer

Chapter 11

Prehabilitation

PHYSICAL REHABILITATION

Physical rehabilitation, or physical therapy helps to improve mobility, function, and quality of life after any illness or surgery. Physical therapy before surgery, called *pre*habilitation, can also improve mobility and speed recovery after surgery. The prehabilitation program consists of eight exercises. Four target your upper body muscles and four work your lower body. These exercises are designed to strengthen typical areas of weakness. You will need an **exercise ball**, a **resistance band**, a **chair**, and a **sturdy table** or **counter** to hold for balance. Your goal is to work up to performing each exercise **15 times** (repetitions) and **3 sets** (of 15 repetitions). Keep track of your progress on an exercise chart such as the one on page 73.

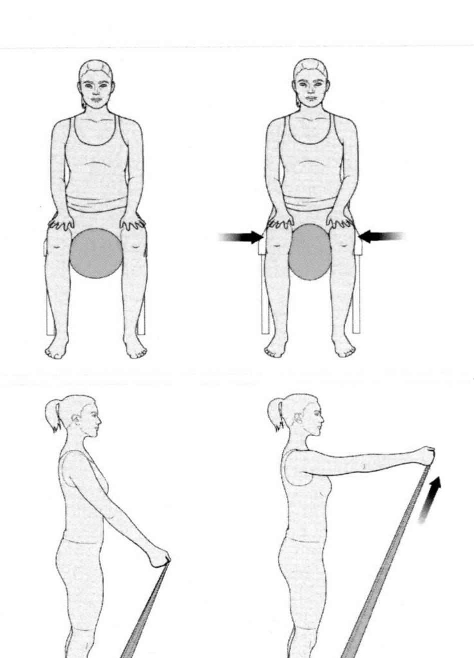

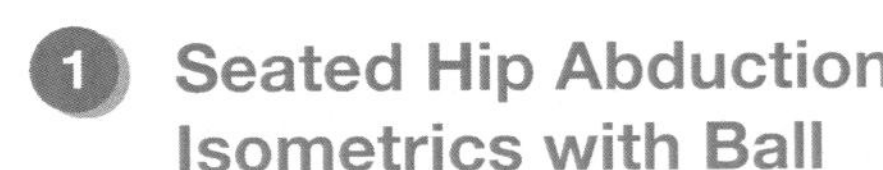

1 Seated Hip Abduction Isometrics with Ball

Position Sit upright on a chair (without arching your back) and place an exercise ball between your legs.

Steps Squeeze both legs together to compress the ball between your knees.

2 Standing Shoulder Flexion with Resistance

Position Stand upright with one end of a resistance band anchored to one foot; hold the other end in your hand.

Steps Lift the arm holding the resistance band straight up to shoulder height and then release slowly to starting position. Repeat with other arm.

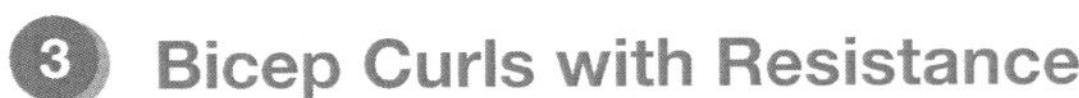

3 Bicep Curls with Resistance

Position Stand upright (without shrugging your shoulders) and with one end of a resistance band anchored to one foot.

Steps Pull up and away while holding the resistance band, bending your elbows.

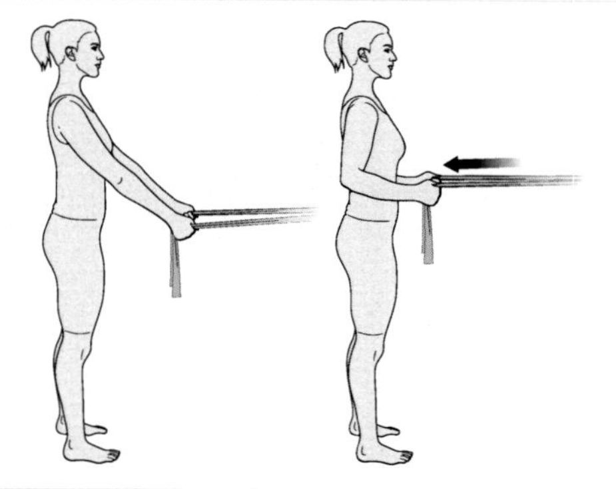

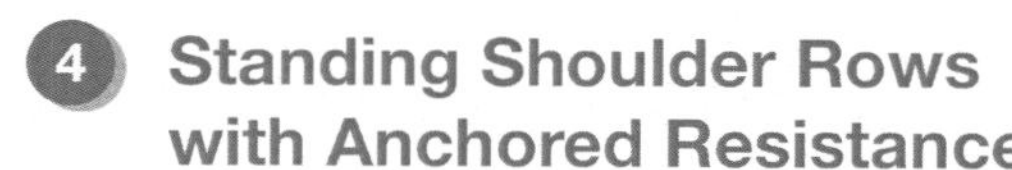

4 Standing Shoulder Rows with Anchored Resistance

Position Stand upright with your back straight and grip the other end of the band with both hands.

Steps Pull your hands backward while holding the resistance band until your elbows reach your sides.

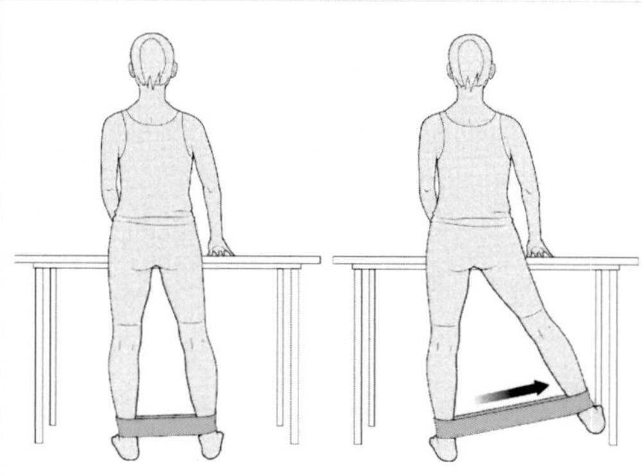

5 Standing Hip Abduction with Resistance at Ankles and Counter Support

Position Stand upright in front of a table or counter with a resistance band looped around your ankles.

Steps Keep one leg straight for balance and lift the other leg sideways against the resistance. Hold for one second and bring back down. Repeat with other leg.

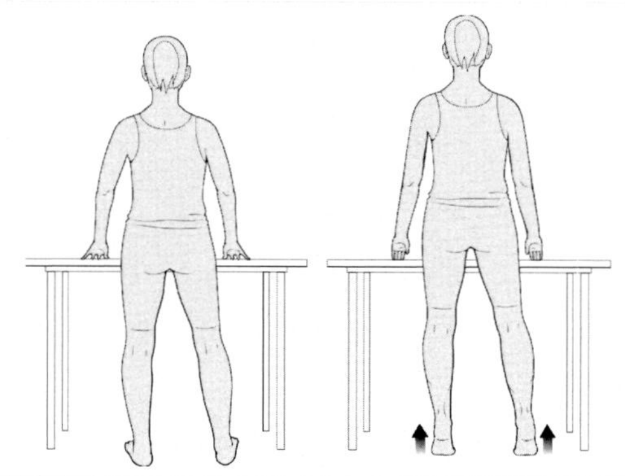

6 Heel Raises with Counter Support

Position Stand upright in front of a table or counter and point feet forward.

Steps Raise your heels off the floor and slowly lower back down.

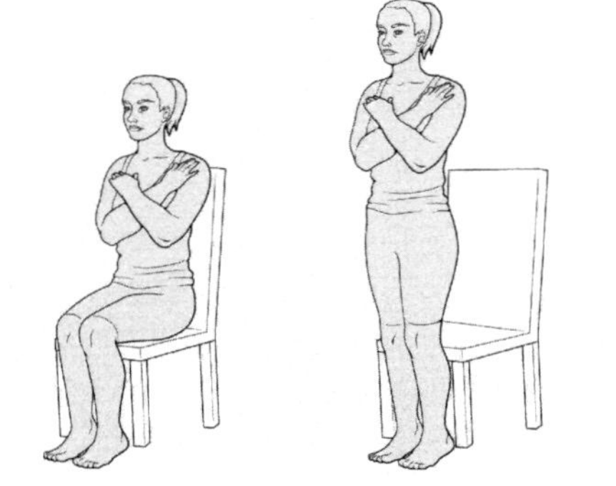

7 Sit to Stand

Position Sit in the middle of a chair and place hands on opposite shoulders. Make sure your back is straight and your feet are flat on the ground. Make sure the chair doesn't move.

Steps Rise to a straight standing position with your arms crossing your chest and then sit back down on the chair.

After Your Surgery

Inpatient exercises
These exercises can be performed right after your surgery and during hospitalization, too. The exercises are based on your limited mobility and pain and are designed to be performed while seated.

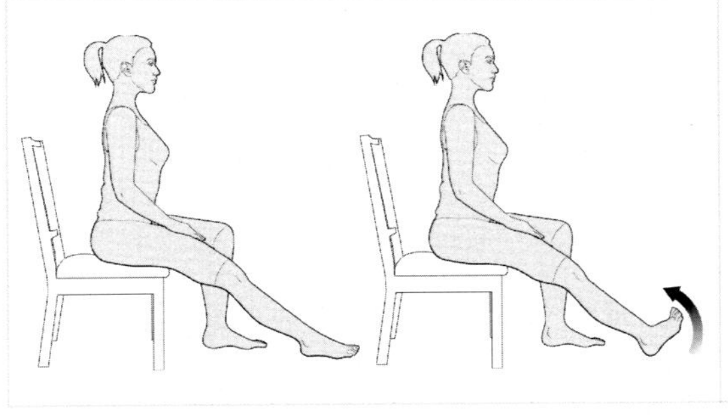

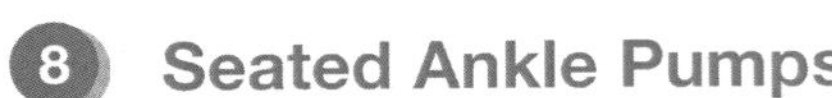

8 Seated Ankle Pumps

Position Sit upright with one leg straight and relaxed.

Steps Bend your foot upward toward you, then point your toes away from you. Repeat with other foot.

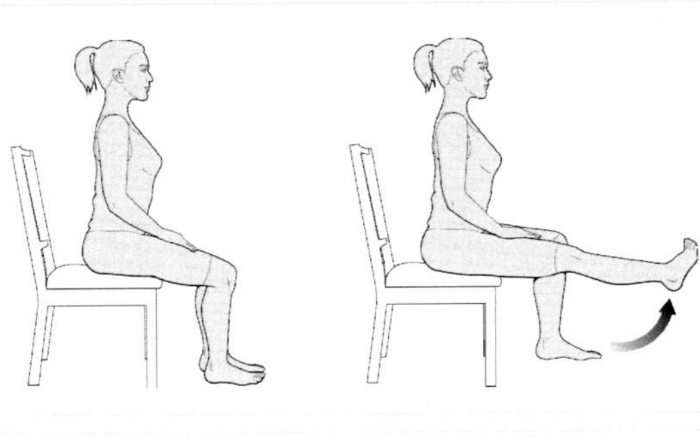

9 Seated Long Arc Quad

Position Sit upright and keep back straight.

Steps Straighten your leg and raise your foot until it is in front of you. Repeat with other leg.

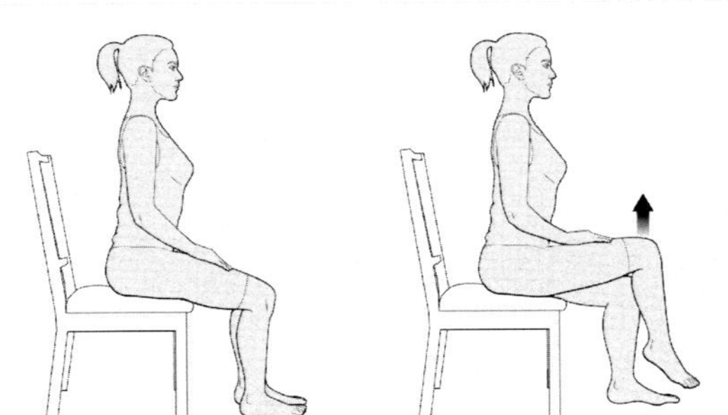

10 Seated March

Position Sit upright and keep back straight.

Steps While knee is bent, lift leg and then lower foot to the floor. Repeat with other foot.

Exercise Log

An example of an exercise log is provided on the next page above.

Instructions
Keep track of your daily exercises in a log. All resistance exercises should be performed three times per week and your sets and repetitions should be recorded for each individual exercise. The goal for each exercise is three sets of 15 repetitions; however, you should complete each workout to your own individual tolerance.

Exercises		Chest Press	Standing Rows	Bicep Curls	Forward Raises	Hip Extension	Hip Abduction	Calf Raises	Sit to Stand
Regimen	MM/DD	3 x 15	3 x 15	3 x 15	3 x 15	3 x 15	3 x 15	3 x 15	3 x 15
Day 1	___/___								
Day 3	___/___								
Day 5	___/___								
Day 7	___/___								
Day 9	___/___								
Day 11	___/___								
Day 13									

Walking Log

Walking is an important part of your prehabilitation. you will be provided with a pedometer to track how many steps you take each day. An example of a walking log is provided below.

Your goal: You should work to increase your steps each day.

Instructions

Wear your pedometer each morning (or if you have a fitbit-type device). Record the number of steps shown on the pedometer screen at the end of the day (right before bed) and then reset. Make sure the pedometer is reset to zero before you begin your day.

Regimen	Day 1	Day 2	Day 3	Day 4	Day 5	Day 6	Day 7	Day 8	Day 9	Day 10	Day 11	Day 12	Day 13	Day 14
Steps	______	______	______	______	______	______	______	______	______	______	______	______	______	______

Chapter 12

Nutrition

WHAT ABOUT MY DIET?

Nutrition is important for cancer treatment and recovery. Proper nutrition can speed recovery and increase your energy and strength. Registered dietitians are experts in nutrition, so if you are having a difficult time with your food intake, seek the services of a dietitian. Most insurance plans will cover this service. Let's take a look at some major components of your food and drink.

Vitamins

Vitamins are vital for many chemical processes in your body. They are obtained mainly through diet and supplements. Animal products, fruits, vegetables, and green leaves are examples of vitamin-rich foods.

Minerals

Minerals are essential for many body functions, including the functioning of your muscles and nerves. Some important minerals are potassium, magnesium, sodium, calcium, chloride, and iron.

Carbohydrates

Carbohydrates are the main energy source for your body and constitute 60% of a healthy diet. Foods such as breads, cereals, fruits, vegetables, and dairy products are rich in carbohydrates.

Simple carbohydrates are those in white and brown sugar, candy, soda and other sweets. **Complex carbohydrates** are fiber and starch, such as those found in whole-grain bread and oatmeal.

Fiber is also found in plant skins, seeds, roots, and even leaves. The more complex the carbohydrate, the better it is for you because complex carbohydrates are packed with more nutrients and are digested more slowly. Fiber-containing nutrients also help regulate your bowel movements and may also reduce your risk of heart disease and diabetes. The recommended daily intake of fiber is 38 grams for men and 25 grams for women.

Fats

Fats are a concentrated source of calories (providing more than twice the energy per gram than carbohydrates and protein). Fats are also an important component of cells. Major sources include meats, dairy products, and oils. Aim to get the majority of your fat intake from monounsaturated fats such as olive and canola oils. Fried and fast foods contain saturated fats and trans fats, which are bad for your health and may increase your risk for heart disease and type 2 diabetes.

Protein

Protein is very important for wound healing. A good way to estimate a three-ounce portion of meat is to use the palm of your hand Quality protein sources include eggs, quinoa (a grain high in protein), milk, yogurt, fish, seafood and tofu.

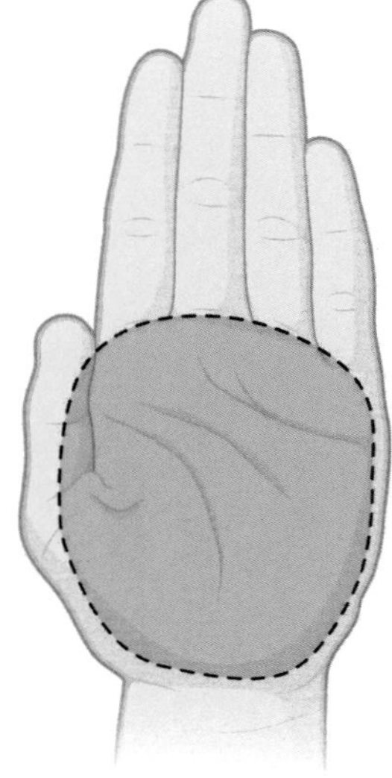

Figure 12.1
The pink circle on the palm is a good approximation of a three-ounce portion of meat.

You should aim for about 0.5 gram of protein per pound of your body weight. Just one egg or one ounce of meat will provide you with seven grams of protein. A typical three-ounce meat sandwich (including the six grams of protein the bread provides) gives you 27 grams of protein!

After surgery, your body will need sufficient protein for healing. You should consume protein throughout the day, especially right before and after physical activity. Remaining physically active and consuming protein will help your muscles receive protein's amino acids for optimal muscle-building.

Foods to Increase Protein Intake

Food	How to use
Hard or semisoft cheese	Melt on muffins, bread, tortillas, meats and fish, vegetables, eggs, stewed fruit, pies and omelets. Grate to include in soups, sauces, casseroles, and vegetables, potato, rice, and noodle dishes.
Cottage cheese and ricotta cheese	Mix with fruits and vegetables. Add into casseroles, noodle dishes, and eggs.
Whole milk	Add to hot and cold cereals, soups, cocoa, puddings, shakes, and smoothies. Use in place of water for cooking and in beverages.
Ice cream and yogurt	Add to milkshakes, desserts, soft or cooked fruit, and smoothies.
Eggs	Add to salads, casseroles, and vegetable dishes. Add extra eggs to omelets, quiches, puddings, custards, and batters.
Nuts, peanut butter, and other nut butters	Finely chop nuts and add to salads or casseroles. Blend with smoothies or shakes. Include nut butters on bread, muffins, fruit and vegetable slices, and ice cream.
Beans, legumes, and tofu	Add to casseroles, soups, pasta and salad dishes, or mash with cheese and milk.
Meat, poultry, and fish	Chop and add to casseroles, soups, salads, sauces, gravies, omelets, quiche, stuffing, and mashed potatoes.

Figure 12.2
Protein intake chart

Food Labels

Food labels are excellent tools for planning a quality diet. Most food packages include food labels, and carbohydrates, fat and protein are listed along with the serving sizes as a percent of the daily recommended value (% Daily Value) per serving.

For example, to your right is a food label fora product with a serving size of one-cup. Note: there are 2 servings per entire container of this product. The one-cup serving provides 250 calories and 18% of the daily recommended value of fat, 10% of the daily total recommended value of carbohydrates, and 20% of the daily recommended value of calcium. This product is a good source of calcium.

Figure 12.3
A simple breakdown of the nutritional facts chart found on most food products.

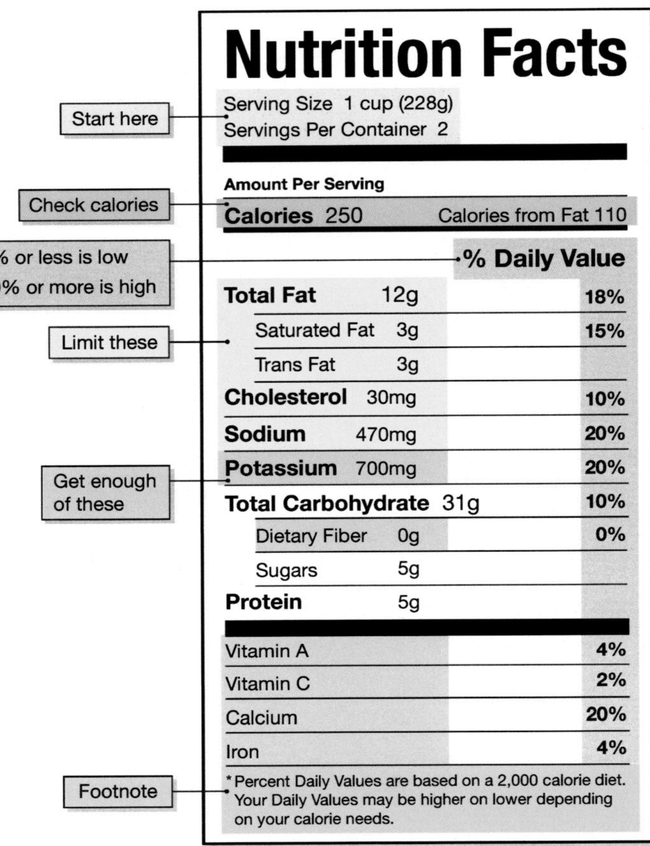

Water and Fluids

Water is the most essential part of our diet and it is involved in nearly every bodily function. Almost all foods contain water, but fruits and vegetables contain the most by weight. You will need more water in hot and/or humid conditions and while you are healing from surgery.

Dehydration

People who undergo bladder removal surgery often suffer from dehydration. This can occur when your fluid intake does not make up for fluid losses that result from normal body function. Signs and symptoms can include dry mouth, fatigue, headache, dizziness, muscle cramps and weakness, irritability, and dark urine.

Dietitians recommend that an individual consumes about **eight glasses of fluid per day** which comes to about about 64 ounces or two liters per day. Fruits are up to 87% water by weight such as apples, pineapple, cranberries, oranges, raspberries, apricots, blueberries and plums. Water-containing vegetables include cucumber, lettuce, zucchini, radish, celery, tomatoes, cabbage, cauliflower, eggplant, peppers, spinach and broccoli.

Poor Appetite Following Surgery

The medications given during surgery slow down the activity of your bowel. Your reduced physical activity following surgery and pain medications both slow digestive activity. This can all contribute to poor appetite and unintentional weight loss. Your body will resort to using fat and muscle stores, which can make you feel more fatigued and prolong this cycle.

Here are some things you can do to enhance your appetite after surgery:

1. **Talk to your medical team**. Untreated nausea or constipation can lead to prolonged poor appetite.

2. **Be physically active as your doctor allows**. Sitting up in a chair or simply walking as you are able after surgery will help to stimulate your appetite.

3. **Try small portions.** Large servings of food can be overwhelming when you are not feeling your best.

4. **Focus on fluids.** When your doctor allows, drinking should be a priority after surgery. If you don't drink enough you may become dehydrated and experience nausea or constipation

5. **A variety of fluids is important**. Water will keep you hydrated, but it won't give you calories, protein, or nutrients (to preserve muscle mass & promote healing). Consider other sources such as broths/ soups for calories and fluid.

6. **For odd tastes in your mouth or dry mouth**, try ice chips, hard candies, lollipops, or Italian Ice. Lemon juice or a slice of citrus fruit in water can quench your thirst, and may taste better.

You should talk to your medical team if you continue to experience poor appetite for a prolonged period despite trying the suggestions listed.

Figure 12.4
Tips on handling food and increasing fuid intake

Food Handling Tips

- Proper food safety when preparing and storing foods is especially important after surgery.
- Wash your hands with hand soap before and after food preparation.
- Rinse vegetables and fruits, including bagged salads, under running water.
- Wash the top of canned goods with soap and water before opening.
- Toss away cracked eggs. Take no chances!
- Use a meat thermometer. Cook meat to 160°F and poultry and reheated leftovers to 165°F.

To Increase Your Fluid Intake

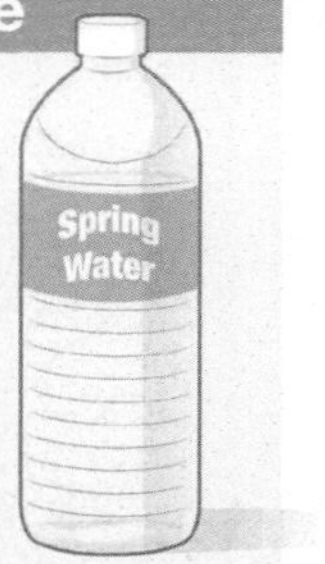

- Fill a 64-ounce (2 liter) water bottle in the morning and drink throughout the day. Emptying the bottle by evening is a good measure of healthy water consumption per day.
- Keep ice chips nearby (a nice diversion from liquid water).
- Enjoy ice pops or Italian ice and keep these in the freezer for convenience.
- Add fruit slices, berries or sliced cucumber to water.

Spring Water

Food Item	Serving Size	Water Content/Serving
Bread	1 slice	0.3 oz (10 ml)
Gelatin (Jell-O)	3.5-oz. snack cup	2 oz (83 ml)
	1 cup	6.5 oz (200 ml)
Ice cream	1 cup	3 oz (100 ml)
Juice	1 cup	7 oz (215 ml)
Watermelon	1 cup	4.5 oz (140 ml)
Yogurt, fruit flavored	6-oz. snack cup	4 oz (126 ml)
	1 cup	6 oz (182 ml)
Chicken, lean, cooked	4 ounces	2 oz (70 ml)
Beef, lean, cooked	4 ounces	2 oz (55 ml)
Grapes	1 cup	4 oz (120 ml)
Banana	1 medium	3 oz (90 ml)
Coffee	4 ounces	6 oz (175 ml)
Tea	4 ounces	5.5 oz (168 ml)

Figure 12.4
Common foods and the amount of water they contain per serving.
A few may surprise you!

Chapter 13

Enhanced Recovery After Surgery (ERAS)

ENHANCED RECOVERY AFTER SURGERY (ERAS)

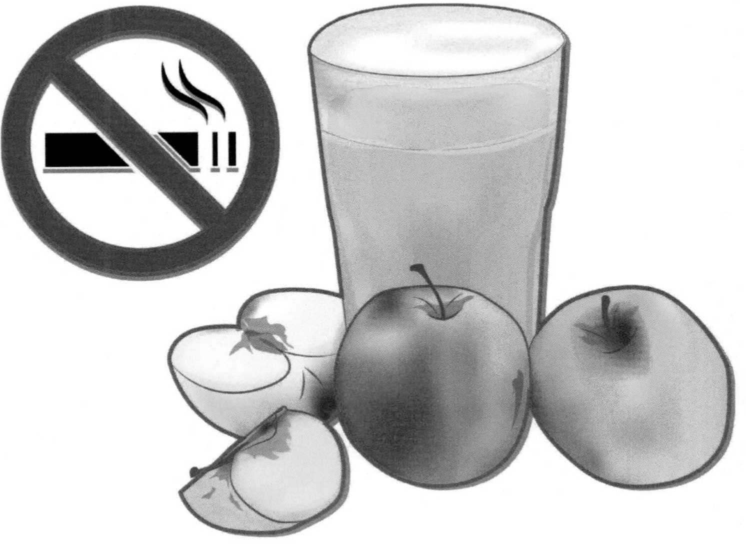

Radical cystectomy is a stressful and complicated procedure. It has negative impacts on both your body and your mind.

Enhanced Recovery After Surgery (ERAS) or "fast track surgery program" is a program that covers all aspects of the patient's care and recovery. ERAS started in the 1990s. It focuses on preparing the patient for surgery with proper counseling and education, improving preoperative health and nutrition, and preventing complications with specific measures and early mobilization.

Studies show that ERAS protocols improve the quality of care, and have been shown to successfully reduce complications, shorten hospital stays and speed return to normal daily activities.

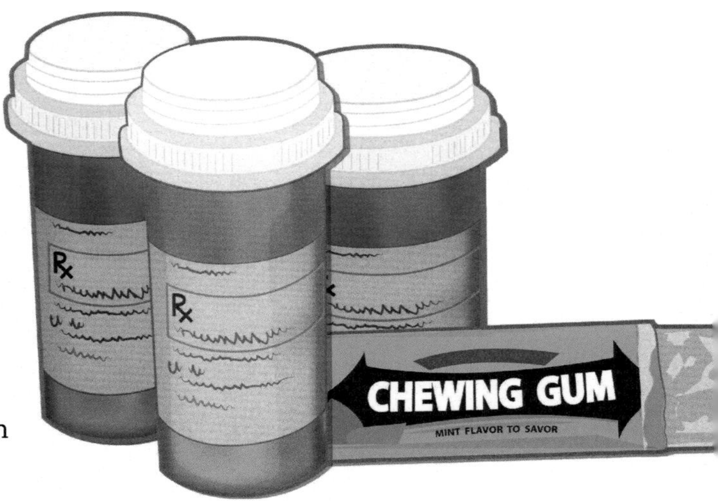

The ERAS program starts on Day One (day of diagnosis or day you decided on surgery), with proper counseling and patient education. Your team (nurses and physicians) will provide a detailed description of the process and what you can expect. Your overall health status will be assessed. A major part of the ERAS program ensures that you are eating well and your body is getting the support it needs.

What the ERAS Pathway Means for You

1 Before Surgery

Patient education and counseling
- Describes the surgery, possible complications and expectations

Preoperative nutrition and health status assessment
- Diet programs with high nutritional values
- Smoking cessation

Physical strength and exercises
- Prehabilitation with home- or office-based exercises

Diet recommendation on the night before the surgery
- Oral intake of fluid rich in complex carbohydrates (apple juice)
- Solid foods allowed up to six hours and liquids up to two hours before surgery

Blood clot prevention
- Compression stockings and anticoagulant medications to avoid formation of clots during the long surgery

2 After Surgery

Early removal of nasogastric tube and promote oral feeding

Attempt removal of urinary catheter at first follow-up visit.

Provide chewing gum to help bowel function return.

Minimize use of pain relievers as tolerated and use drugs to avoid nausea and vomiting.

Early mobilization and walking as soon as the first day. Prehabilitation improves early mobilization.

Early return to eating, as tolerated by the patient.

Discharge criteria
- Adequate pain control
- Regular diet
- Normal bowel function
- Competence in stoma care (ileal conduit)

Chapter 14

What Is a Quality Operation?

ASSESSING THE QUALITY OF SURGERY

TURBT

A quality TURBT procedure means:

- Any visible tumor was completely removed.
- The removed tissue includes muscle in the specimen to be able to properly stage the disease.
- No perforation of the bladder wall.
- Bleeding is fully controlled before completion of procedure.

Radical Cystectomy

Radical cystectomy is a major surgical procedure that may last up to seven hours and includes removal of multiple organs in addition to construction of urinary diversion. Even with the best surgeon, radical cystectomy has been shown to have a high complication rate (40% - 60%), with 1% possibility of death at 30 days, and 5% within 90 days after surgery.

Several key quality indicators can lead to better outcomes of this complex procedure. At Roswell Park Cancer Institute, we have developed and tested quality criteria: the Quality Cystectomy Score. The quality criteria are measured from the time you decide to have surgery up to 30 days after surgery. It is wise to discuss these quality measures with your surgeon.

QUALITY MEASURES

Preoperative (Before Surgery)

Neoadjuvant Chemotherapy
Ask your surgeon whether you are eligible for chemotherapy before surgery (also called neoadjuvant chemotherapy). Having chemotherapy before surgery helps to get rid of cancer cells that may spread to other areas but cannot be seen on scans. Studies show that patients who have neoadjuvant chemotherapy have up to 6% - 8% better survival. You may not be eligible, but discuss this option with your surgeon and medical oncologist.

Operative

Shorter Surgery
This is a long, complex operation with multiple steps. The quality cystectomy score uses six and a half hours as a cut off time. Surgeries that can be completed in less than six and a half hours are best.

Limited Blood Loss
Estimated blood loss is kept to less than 500 ml.

Pathologic

Negative Surgical Margins
Once this surgery is completed, your bladder and other removed tissues should show negative surgical margins. Surgical margins are the edges of the tissue removed, which are checked for any disease left behind.

Adequate Lymph Node Removal
A thorough removal of the lymph nodes is critical. (Refer to Chapter 8). Ideally, more

than 20 nodes should be removed. However this can vary depending on your individual anatomy or how the pathology was conducted.

Post-operative (After Surgery)

This is the time from surgery to initial recovery. Any death, readmission to the hospital or high-grade complication that which needs intervention is considered a negative quality indicator. Complications happen during radical cystectomy, but managing them well is the key to recovery.

Patients are assigned a star score based on the number of criteria achieved.

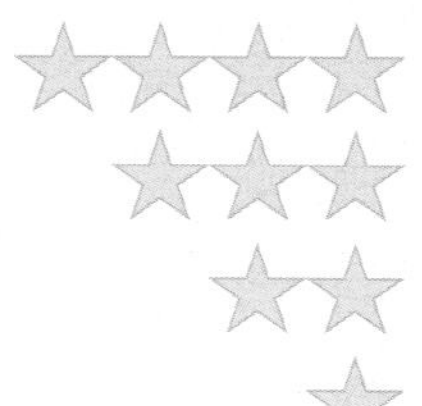

4 star - 7 or 8 criteria met

3 star - 5 or 6 criteria met

2 star - 3 or 4 criteria met

1 star - 1 or 2, or any mortality within 30 days of surgery

Quality Cystectomy Score has been shown to be a good indicator of cancer control and survival after surgery. Patients who achieve a higher score (3 or 4 stars) have better cancer control and live longer.

After your surgery, talk to your doctor about your QCS and discuss your next steps.

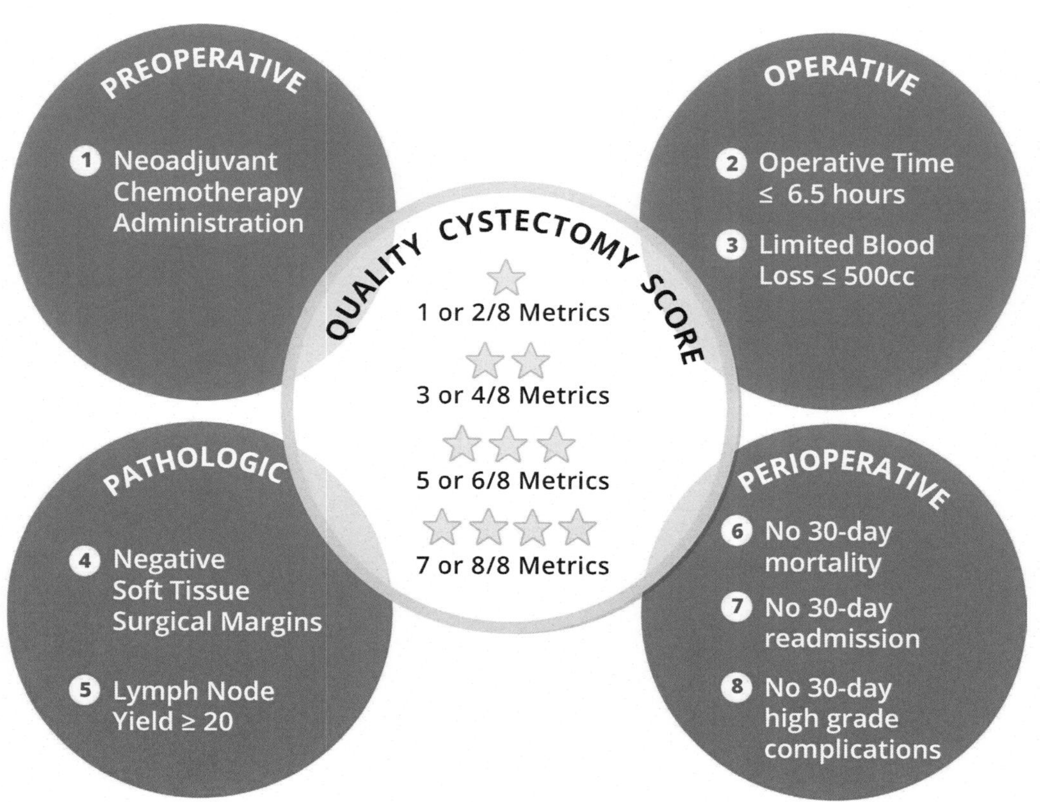

Chapter 15

Neoadjuvant Chemotherapy

NEOADJUVANT CHEMOTHERAPY

Your physician may recommend chemotherapy before your surgery. This is known as "neoadjuvant chemotherapy" (NAC). Giving chemotherapy before surgery aims to shrink the tumor and kill any cancer cells outside the bladder that might remain after surgery.

Recent studies have shown that NAC can improve survival in patients undergoing cystectomy for bladder cancer, without increased risks or complications. Shrinking the tumor before surgery can make it easier for your surgeon to remove all the cancer.

Who Can Have NAC?

Patients whose cancer is confined to the bladder, who have adequate kidney function and hearing and have no severe nerve damage, may be candidates for NAC. (Cisplatin, the most powerful chemotherapy for bladder cancer, can damage the kidneys.)

What Drugs Are Used?

- **Cisplatin-based combination chemotherapy**
  The two most commonly-used drug regimens are MVAC (methotrexate, vinblastine, adriamycin and cisplatin) and GC (gemcitabine and cisplatin). These two regimens are about the same in terms of how well they kill cancer, but some studies favor GC, because it may be better tolerated.

- **Classic MVAC**
  This combines Methotrexate, Vinblastine, h, and Cisplatin administered every 28 days for three cycles. Each cycle is given on a period of four days: Day 1, 2, 15 and 22.

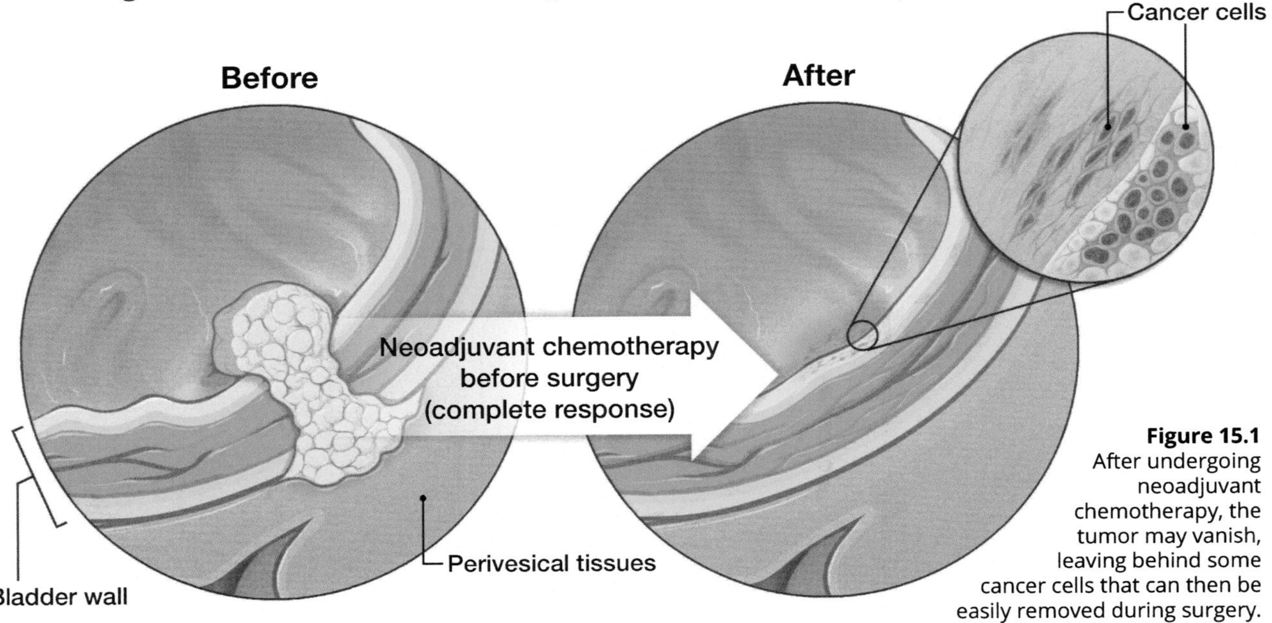

Figure 15.1
After undergoing neoadjuvant chemotherapy, the tumor may vanish, leaving behind some cancer cells that can then be easily removed during surgery.

- **Dose dense MVAC**
  This increases the intensity of the treatment by administering it every 14 days with G-CSF (a growth factor) for three to four cycles. Dose-dense neoadjuvant regimen is a recent approach, with promising results of improved disease-free survival and high compliance.

- **GC**
  GC combines Gemcitabine and Cisplatin, given every 28 days for a maximum of six cycles. Each cycle is a period of four days; day 1, 2, 8 and 15.

- **CMV**
  This combines Methotrexate, Vinblastine and Cisplatin, repeated every 28 days for three cycles.

Patients with abnormal kidney function, impaired hearing, neuropathy or poor health status should not receive cisplatin. Your physician may prescribe another less-toxic drug called carboplatin. Such regimens are less effective and are not recommended by most guidelines. NAC is also not advised for people who are unlikely to tolerate at least three cycles of chemotherapy.

How Does NAC Work?

NAC works in two ways. It shrinks the tumor in the bladder and controls and eliminates cancer cells that have escaped the bladder but cannot be seen on scans (micro-metastatic disease). Chemotherapy is beneficial in approximately 70% of the patients who are treated.

What Are the Advantages?

The biggest benefit of chemotherapy is the likelihood of increasing cure rates in bladder cancer. On average, NAC prior to surgery improves survival by up to 10%. However, the benefit may be even higher (up to 40% increase in cure rates) in patients where chemotherapy eliminates most of the cancer prior to surgery. Surgery is still essential, and NAC improves the results of surgery but does not replace it. NAC does not increase the risk of complications associated with surgery.

Are There Side Effects?

NAC, like any chemotherapy that circulates throughout the body, is effective at targeting cancer cells. Unfortunately, these powerful drugs may also affect normal tissues, including:

1. Kidneys (for cisplatin)
2. Bone marrow, especially the manufacture of blood cells responsible for fighting infections, clotting and carrying oxygen in the blood
3. Skin cells and hair follicles, causing hair loss
5. Gastrointestinal tract, causing nausea and vomiting
6. Nerve cells, causing neuropathy (numbness and tingling and hearing loss (especially cisplatin)
7. Heart failure (especially adriamycin)

NAC does not work with some types of bladder cancer, such as squamous cell carcinoma and adenocarcinoma. To date there is no way to know which patients will respond to NAC.

Therefore, not all patients will benefit from it. Some patients may suffer complications associated with the chemotherapy without real benefit. Also, non-responders may have their surgery delayed without real benefit from NAC, which may then adversely affect their outcome. You must discuss these potential outcomes with your physician team when choosing the best treatment for you.

Chapter 16

Taking My Bladder Out

TAKING MY BLADDER OUT

Cystectomy

A cystectomy is a surgery where the doctor removes your entire bladder. Ideally, all of the cancer is removed with the bladder.

What happens during the procedure?
It's helpful to understand your urinary tract to understand this procedure. You have one kidney on each side of your body. Your kidneys filter blood, making urine.

Tubes called ureters connect your kidneys to your bladder, which empties through your urethra (See Chapter 3).

During the surgery, the doctor first cuts the ureters. Next, the front of your bladder is separated from the abdominal wall. Then, the urethra is cut. Your bladder – now freed – can be removed. To ensure that all the cancer is eliminated adjacent organs may also be removed (prostate in men, and uterus, cervix and portion of vagina in women). Because you no longer have a bladder, the doctor creates a place for your urine to be stored. In a later chapter on urinary diversion, you will learn more about how this is done.

What makes this surgery "radical"?
A radical surgery tries to get all of the disease–the cancer–by taking nearby organs and tissues in addition to the organ with the cancer.

In a cystectomy, "radical" refers to removing: (1) the entire bladder with adjacent organs (prostate in men), (2) nearby lymph nodes, (3) sometimes the urethra, and (4) some of the reproductive organs. The removed reproductive organs may include:

- Prostate (men)
- Uterus (women)
- Ovaries (women)
- Vagina (women)

These organs are taken out because they are too close to the bladder. Sometimes the cancer spreads to them but remains too small to see. Removing them can help prevent your cancer from returning.

How will this operation affect my life?
Radical cystectomy is a major surgery which permanently changes your body, including how you will urinate and preserve your sexual abilities.

How you urinate after surgery depends on the method of urinary diversion you and your doctor decided upon.

Two Ways to Replace the Job of Your Bladder:

1. **Outside your body:**
   The doctor creates a hole in your abdomen-called a stoma–for your urine to come through. Your urine will be collected in a bag outside your body, which you will wear close to your belly.
2. **Inside your body:**
   A replacement bladder (or neobladder) within your body is created from the small intestine to store your urine. It may be connected to either your urethra or to a catheterizable opening. Both versions of this may require using a catheter, to be inserted into the replacement bladder to empty it. These are permanent changes that mean a major adjustment. Counseling services and

support groups are very helpful to patients with bladder cancer.

Most patients are able to adjust, adapt to these changes, and live a happy life after surgery. Your doctor's job is to help you understand your surgery and what changes to expect and to help you decide what is right for you.

For Men

Male cystectomy

A male cystectomy usually means removing the prostate, too. Your prostate sits directly below the bladder, where the urethra connects to the bladder. The prostate may contain some bladder cancer cells because it is so close, and may allow the cancer to come back.

Figure 16.2
Side view of the organs removed during a male cystectomy and urethrectomy

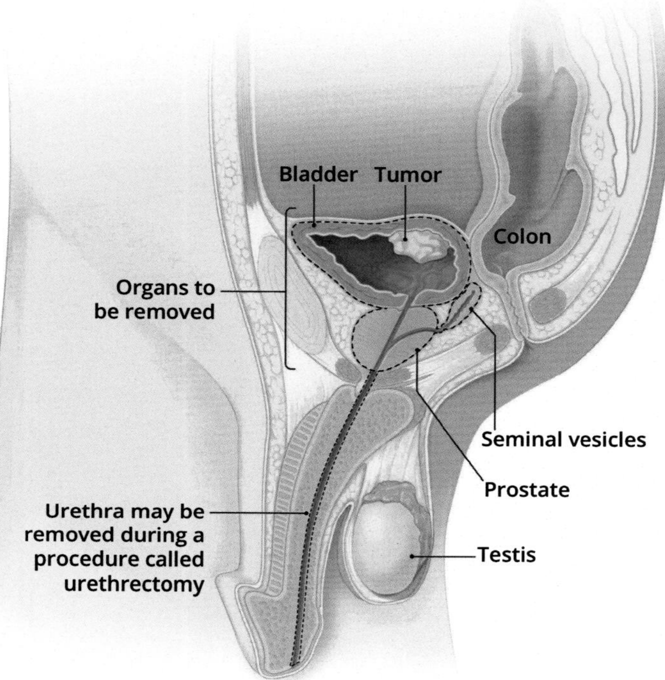

Figure 16.1
Posterior view of prostate with urethra and adjacent nerves

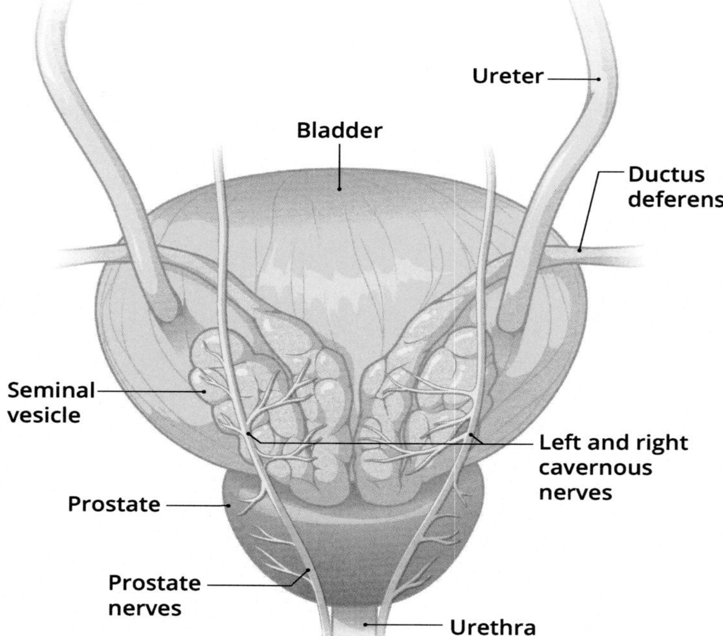

Prostate cancer is also very common in older men. For these reasons, the prostate is almost always removed in a radical cystectomy. In some patients, it's possible to spare the prostate, but it's risky and provides few benefits. Your doctor will help direct you to the best treatment plan for you and your diagnosis.

Will I be able to have sex?

Most men who have a radical cystectomy have trouble with sexual function. Erections are controlled by nerves that travel on the surface of the prostate, just below the bladder. Sometimes doctors can avoid damaging these nerves, but unfortunately it is often unavoidable. Some options, such as a penile implant or prescription medications inserted into the urethra or shaft of the penis, can restore sexual function after surgery. If this is a concern, you must discuss it with your doctor. Together you can come up with a plan that best suits you.

For Women

Female Cystectomy

You may hear your surgeon refer to this procedure as "anterior pelvic exenteration." This means that your reproductive organs–uterus, ovaries, fallopian tubes, and part of the vagina–are removed along with your bladder and urethra. Your surgeon removes these organs to minimize the chance that your cancer comes back. In addition, the lymph nodes near your bladder are also removed.

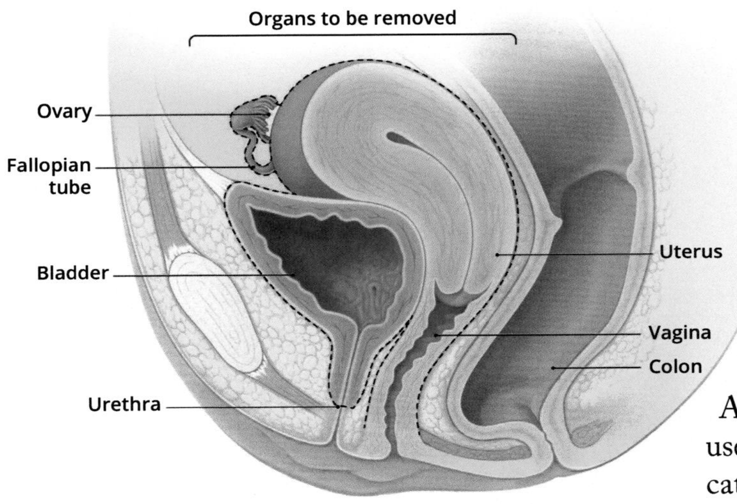

Figure 16.3
Side view of the organs removed during a female cystectomy & urethrectomy.

Why must my reproductive organs be removed if I only have bladder cancer?

The uterus (or womb) touches the top and back of your bladder, and bladder cancer may spread–or metastasize–to it. Other female reproductive organs–ovaries, cervix, and vagina–may be at risk because they are located near your bladder. Some women may be eligible for reproductive organ sparing procedures, which means select reproductive organs are not removed.

Your doctor will advise you on what type of procedure you should have depending on your age and your risk of the cancer spreading or recurring. This risk depends on:

- Location of your tumor
- Aggressiveness (stage and grade) of your cancer

For example, if your cancer is located on the back of your bladder, there may be greater risk to the reproductive organs. If the tumor has already spread outside of your bladder (stage T3), the surgeon will need to remove all of the female reproductive organs.

Do I need to have my urethra removed?

The decision to remove your urethra, the tube that allows you to empty urine from your body, depends on the location of the tumor in your bladder.

A procedure called an ileal conduit may be used to release urine from your body. Or a catheterizable pouch (you will self-catheterize) may be used. (More on this in Chapters 17 and 18).

If part of my vagina is removed, will I still be able to have sexual intercourse?

Removing the front part of your vagina may affect sexual function. If you need your vagina removed, your surgeon may be able to rebuild it using various surgical techniques.

What happens if my uterus is removed?
If you have not reached menopause, you will no longer get your period and you will not be able to get pregnant.

If you have gone through menopause, your uterus is not functional and its removal will not lead to side effects. In addition, the removal of your uterus will eliminate your risk for uterine cancer.

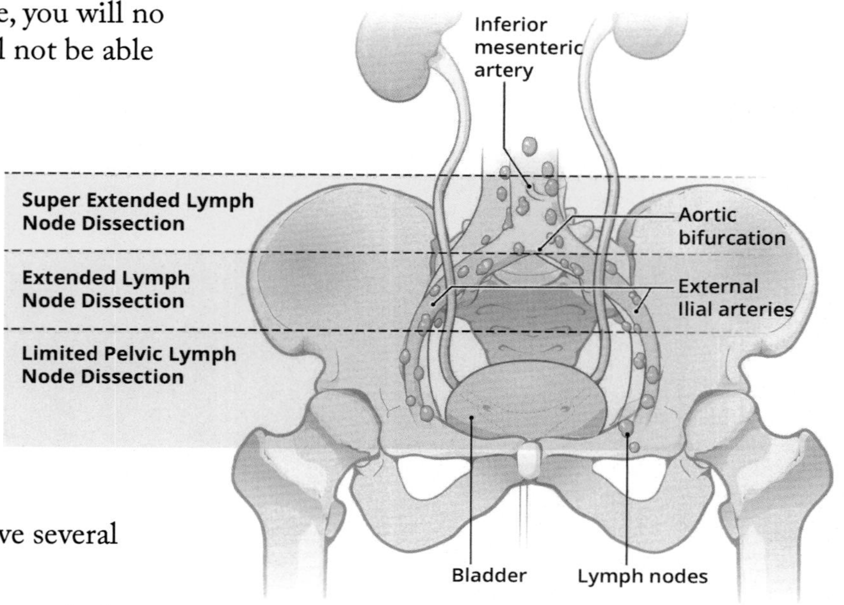

Figure 16.4
Three levels of lymph node dissection

What happens if my ovaries are removed?
Before menopause, your ovaries have several functions:

- The ovary releases an egg each month that may be fertilized, leading to pregnancy.
- The ovary produces female hormones (body chemicals that control many body functions).

If you have not reached menopause, removing the ovaries may lead to an early menopause. On the other hand, if you have reached menopause, you will experience fewer side effects. For all women, the risk of ovarian cancer is eliminated following removal of the ovaries.

Lymph Node Removal

Every radical cystectomy must also include removing nearby lymph nodes, because bladder cancer may have spread to them. Most surgeons recommend an extended lymph node dissection (removal) shown below in the blue shaded area. A thorough lymph node removal means improved survival. Make sure you and your surgeon discuss removing lymph nodes as part of your surgical procedure.

Lymphedema

Lymph is a protein-rich fluid present all over the body like a drainage system. Lymphedema is observed when lymph accumulates after the removal of lymph nodes, because all those channels of drainage are disrupted. Lymph can build up in areas such as the scrotum and lower legs. Symptoms may include heaviness of feet or scrotum and stretching of the skin. Lymphedema can be managed by elevating the legs or by wearing compression stockings. The condition usually improves within 6 weeks of surgery. If it persists a lymphedema clinic is dedicated to help with different options to improve quality of life.

Comparing Robot Assisted Surgery to Open Surgery

Robot-assisted Surgery

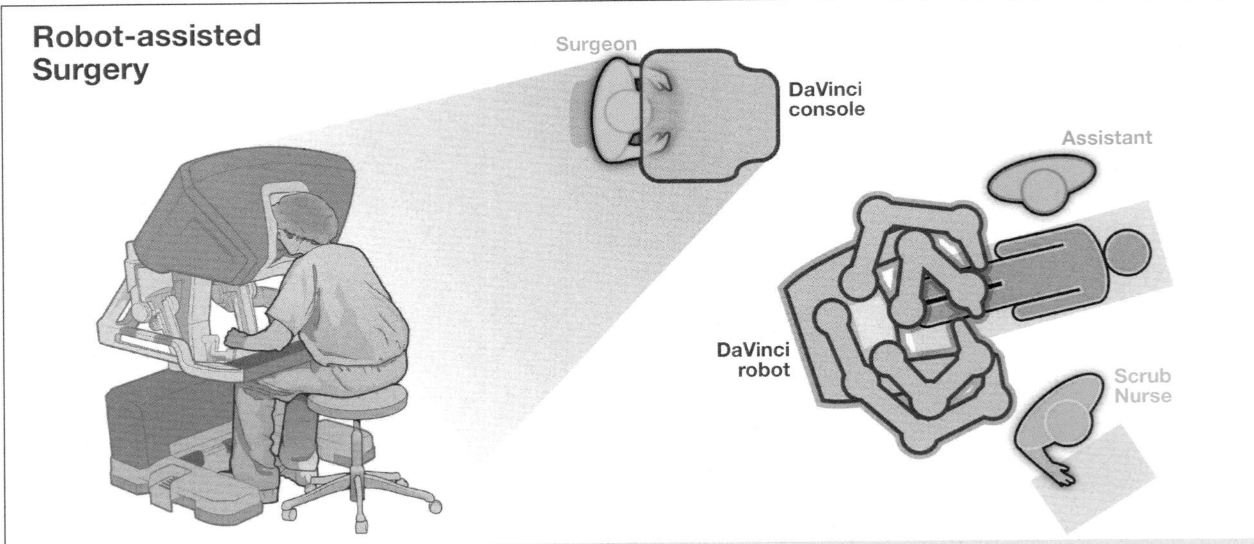

- Robot-assisted surgery is the modern twist on traditional surgery using advanced technology.
- Robots do not perform surgery.
- Surgeon is placed away from patient
- The robot assists the surgeon.
- Advantages: gives surgeon 3D vision, magnifies operative field 10X, uses minituarized tools and hands with greater freedom of movement

Open Traditional Surgery

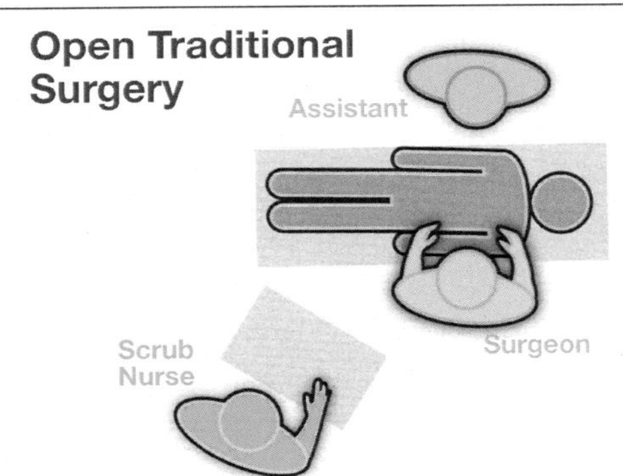

- Surgeon remains next to patient
- Traditional method of performing surgery
- Advantage: surgeons can touch and feel the tissue in the operative field
- Disadvantage: bigger incision, greater blood loss

**In both surgeries, the most important factor is the experience of the surgeon. Always ask about your surgeon's experience in the procedure you are undergoing.*

Chapter 17

Ileal Conduit and Stoma Care

ILEAL CONDUIT (UROSTOMY)

If your cancer is too close to your urethra, where urine passes out of the body, or your kidneys are unable to handle the stress, then it may not be safe for your surgeon to create a neobladder for you. If this happens, you may undergo an ileal conduit with urostomy.

What is an ileal conduit?
After removing your bladder, your surgeon will remove a small piece (about 15cm) of your small intestine called an 'ileum'. One end of the ileum will be connected to your ureters (tubes from the kidneys) and the other end will be brought out through the abdomen, and a stoma will be created. Finally, your intestine will be reconnected.

Urostomy

- With urostomy, your surgeon makes a route for urine to pass out of your body through a new opening in your skin near the belly button.
- This route connects the tubes from your kidneys (ureters) to the new opening near your belly button. This opening is called a stoma or ostomy.
- A special bag that covers this opening collects your urine and acts as your new bladder.
- Whenever the bag gets full, you will empty the same way you used to empty your bladder.

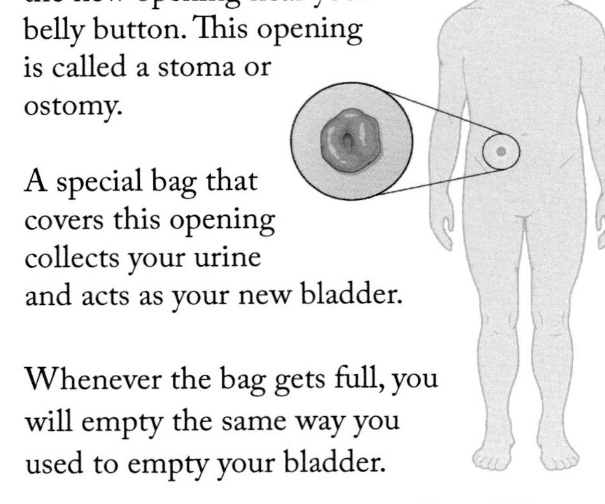

Figure 17.2
Zoomed-in view of the stoma

What is a stoma?
A stoma is another word for an opening to the body. Your urine goes through the ileum (piece of bowel) and out your body through the stoma, a small opening near your belly button.

Figure 17.1
After the bladder is removed, it may be replaced by an ileal conduit.

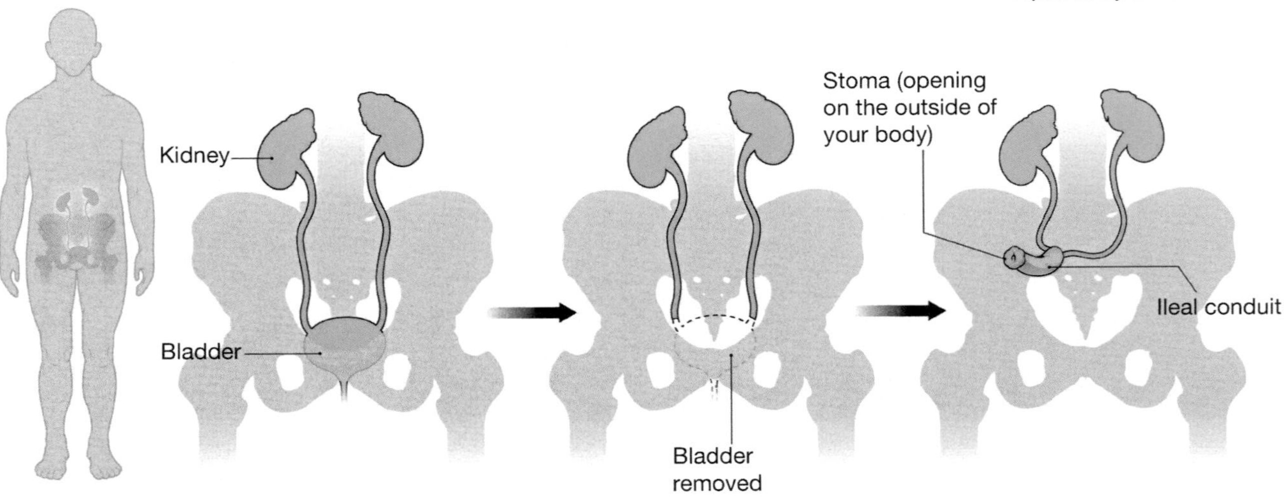

Before the operation

You will meet with a stoma care nurse, who will go over the surgery and tell you what to expect during your hospital stay and when you return home. Doctors will mark a site on your abdomen for the opening of your stoma. The site will be a few inches from your belly button, but away from your waistline and other body creases and folds to help ensure your stoma will not interfere with everyday activities.

After the operation

A bag placed on top of your stoma will collect your urine. For two weeks after your surgery, two tubes (stents) will come from the stoma. These tubes are attached to the kidneys and help you to heal properly. These tubes will either fall out into your pouch or your doctor will remove them. (This is not a painful procedure). After the operation, your stoma care nurse will help you learn to care for your stoma and become independent and comfortable.

Why do I need a bag over my stoma?

The stoma is an opening; it cannot store urine. Therefore, a small amount of urine will always flow out the stoma. In order to keep urine from constantly leaking out of your body, a bag over your stoma collects the urine flowing. A sticky patch on the bag helps it stick to the skin on your abdomen.

When will the bag be put on?

After you wake up from the operation, the bag will already be in place on your stoma. The small tubes coming out of it will be removed as you recover. During these first days after the operation, the bag will be changed by hospital staff and they will help you learn how to do it yourself.

Figure 17.3
A more detailed view of how an ileal conduit is formed

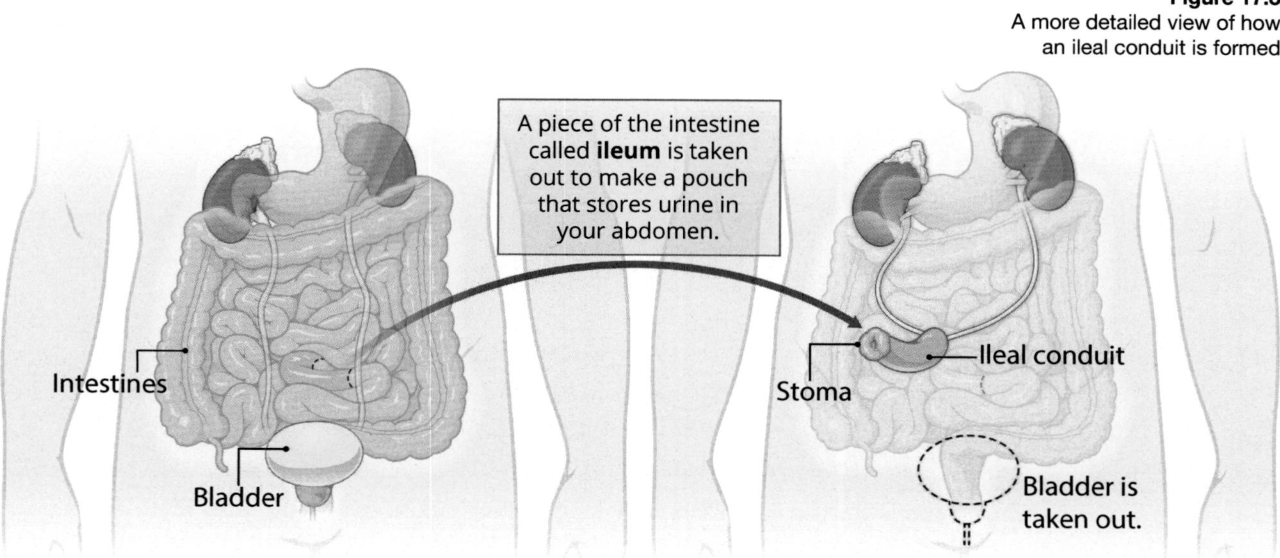

Is this bag forever?
Yes, you will have to use this bag for the rest of your life. It is important to understand its function, how to replace it and cope with other problems that may occur.

How is the bag fixed to it?
The stoma cover has two parts: (1) The sticky patch and (2) the bag. The sticky patch is cut to fit around your stoma and attaches to the skin around the stoma. It can be peeled off your skin easily. The bag is positioned over the stoma and attached to the sticky patch to cover it completely. A small spout at the end of the bag allows you to empty the bag as you need to. (It locks!)

I don't think I can do this on my own!
Yes, you can! Initially, most people need help changing the bag. In the hospital, nursing staff will do it and when you go home, a family member can help you. Over the next couple of months, caring for your stoma and changing the bag will get easier and you will learn to do it yourself.

How do I change the bag?
Refer to Figures 17.4 and 17.5 for a list of supplies you need and the steps to follow to change your stoma bag.

How do I get my stoma supplies?
You will be given a prescription for your supplies, which you can take to a supplier. (You will be given a list of suppliers after your surgery.) Call ahead to make sure the suppliers carry your ostomy supplies. Some suppliers offer home delivery.

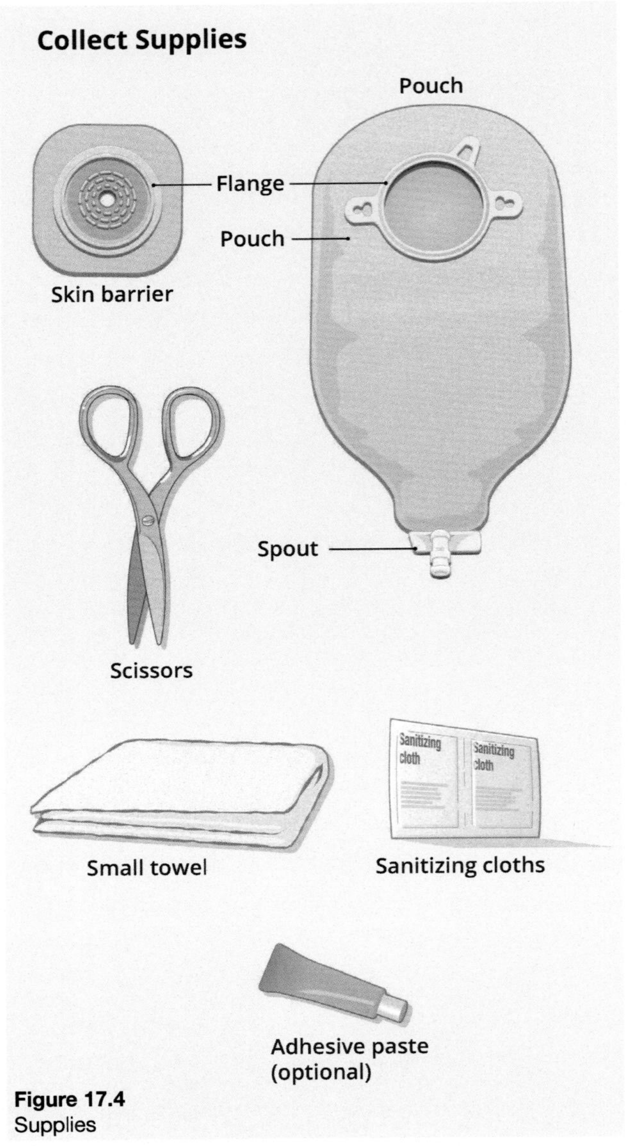

Figure 17.4
Supplies

How often do I need to change the bag?
It varies. Just after surgery, you may need to change the bag more often (as it may fall off or leak). Once you become experienced, it can stay attached to your skin for four to seven days. Throughout the day, you may empty your urine bag every two to three hours. At night, you can use a larger bag so you won't have to wake during the night to empty it. Your night bag should be replaced every month, and you must

Steps for Changing Your Stoma Bag

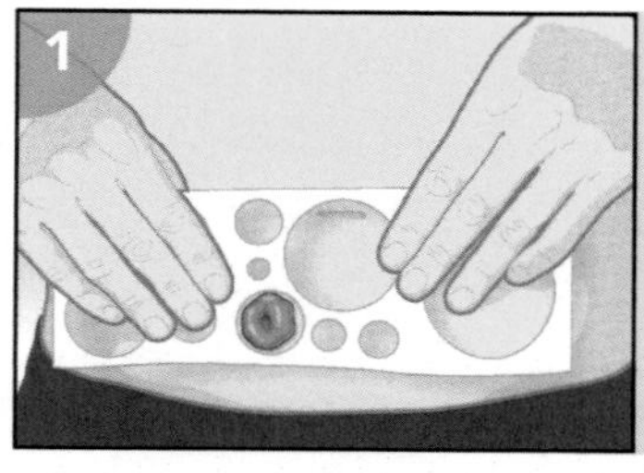

Use the sizing guide to identify the stoma diameter

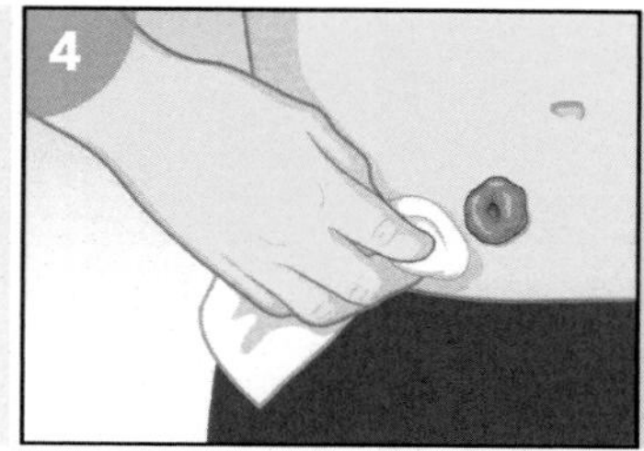

Clean your skin with soap and water

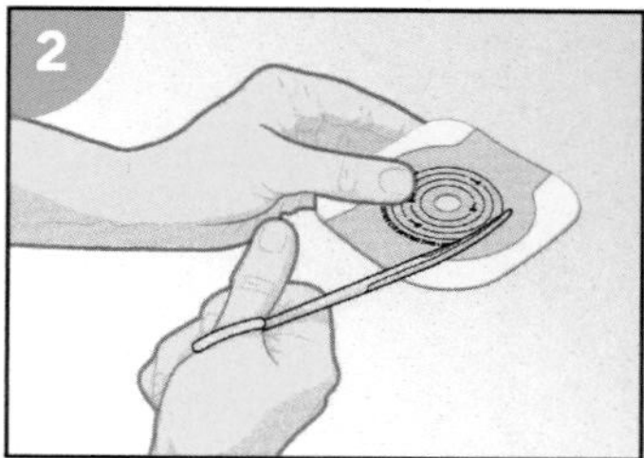

Cut an opening in the skin barrier to match the size of your bag's flange

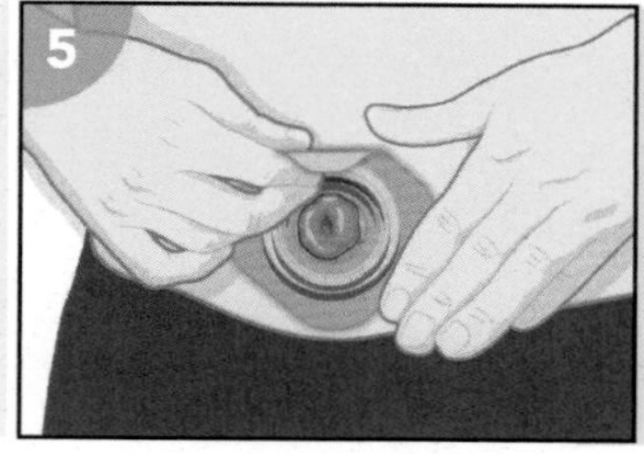

Apply skin barrier over the stoma

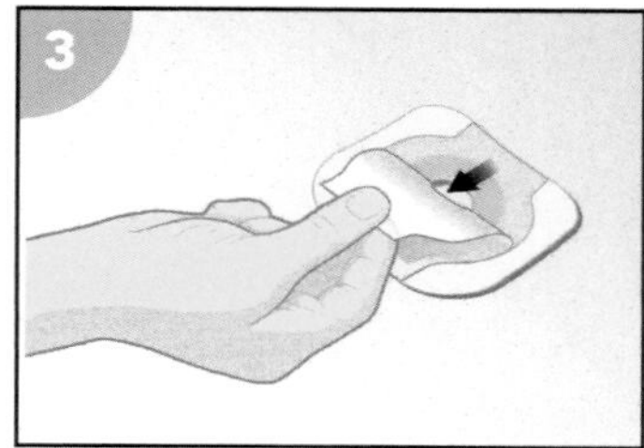

Remove the adhesive cover leave face up

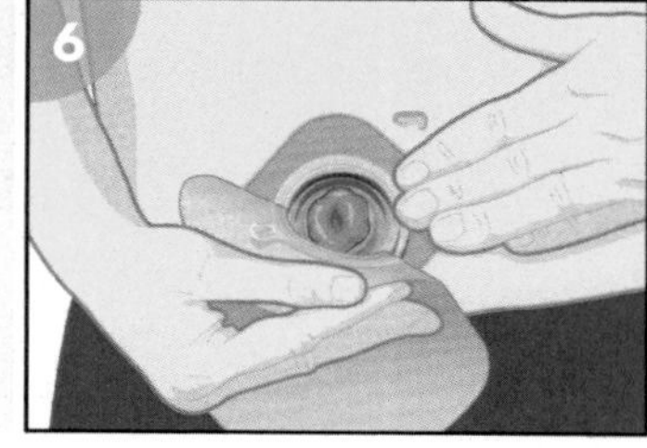

Attach pouch to skin barrier. Ensure the bag is secured

Figure 17.5

rinse it weekly (or daily) with a solution of equal parts vinegar and water.

How do I empty the bag?
Each bag has a lock on the bottom. When the lock is opened, urine will empty (Figure 17.6).

1. Sit on the toilet.
2. Hold the lock and gently unlock it.
3. Direct the flow of urine into the toilet.
4. When empty, lock securely and dry the end with a tissue.
5. Wash your hands after handling the bag.

Make sure that you empty the bag when it is a little over half filled. Waiting for it to fill completely will create a pull on the patch, and it may fall off.

Do's and Don'ts

- Do clean or wipe with gentle strokes.
- Don't rub the stoma (never!)
- Do use clean water to wash the stoma.
- Don't use hot water.
- Don't wear tight belts or large belt buckles over or near your stoma.
- Do continue to drink a healthy amount of fluids. Don't avoid fluids in the hope that you will empty your bag less often.

I used to be pretty active. Can I still do my normal activities?
Yes, you can perform all normal activities, such

Figure 17.6
Different ways of emptying the bag

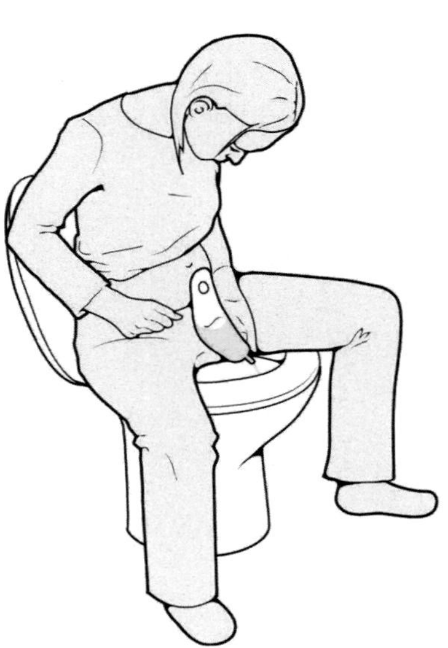
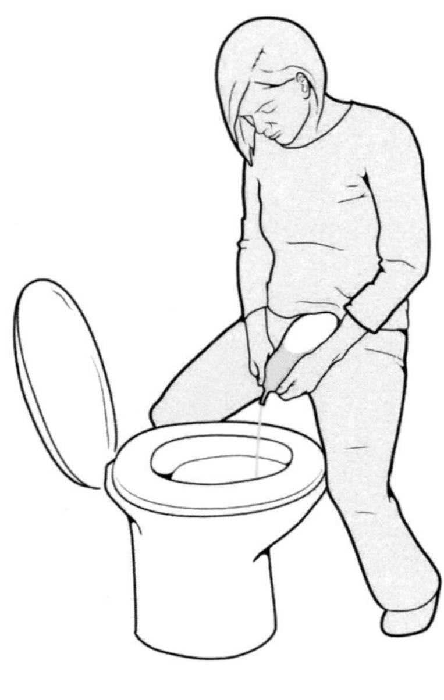
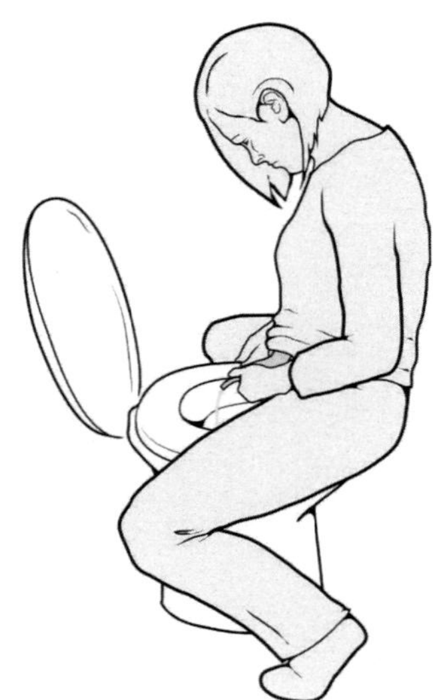

as gardening, jogging, non-strenuous sports and even swimming.

Avoid rough contact sports such as football. You can shower with the bag on or off, but avoid direct jets of water on your stoma. Always empty your bag before you start these activities. Always keep a bag with all your stoma supplies with you at the gym, work, or if you go out, just in case you need to change your bag.

Can I have sex with the stoma and bag?
Yes, the stoma and bag should not interfere with your close relationships. Make sure you empty the bag before having sex. Opaque covers are available that hide the bag and its contents. You can also purchase garments made specifically for people with ostomies.

Can I still go on vacation with my stoma?
Yes, having a stoma should not prevent you from normal daily activities. Plan ahead for travel. Carry twice the amount of supplies you normally need on your flight. Place your seatbelt over or under the stoma. Make sure you have contacts for stoma suppliers at your destination.

Will I have any side effects from my stoma?
You may have some side effects with your stoma, or problems related to securing the sticky patch and bag.

- **Skin irritation**
  The skin around your stoma may become irritated or develop a rash. Take care to prevent urine from leaking onto your skin and keep the skin under the patch dry. If you get a rash, apply special paste to help soothe it. (Figure 17.7).

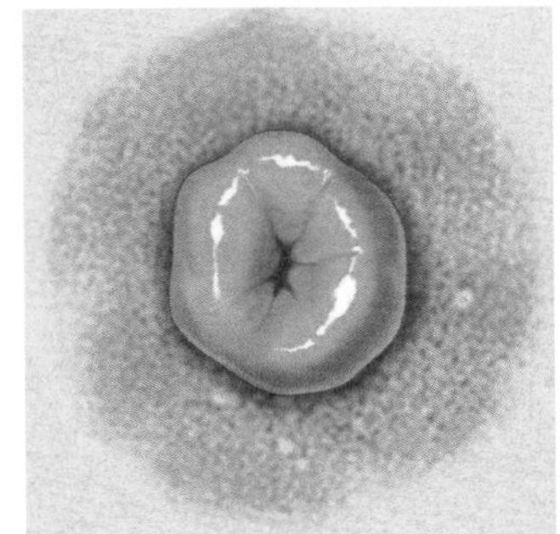

Figure 17.7
Red, irritated skin around the stoma

- **Dehydration**
  Because the stoma is made from the bowel, you may lose body fluid and have changes to your body's salt levels. Prevent dehydration by drinking adequate fluids, including water, fruit juices or Gatorade. (Refer to Chapter 12 on Nutrition)

- **Urinary tract infection**
  A urinary tract infection is the most common side effect of having a stoma. Prevent infections by drinking enough water and keeping your stoma clean and healthy.

- **Hernia**
  Over time, your stoma may develop a small hernia (bulging mass). Abdominal hernias are common because your muscles are weakened by surgery. Use proper lifting methods to avoid straining your abdominal muscles. If you develop a hernia, your doctor can prescribe a hernia support belt or can repair the hernia through surgery. (Figure 17.8).

- **Fallen stoma**
  Your stoma may lose its shape or sink back into your skin. This may increase your risk for a skin rash around your stoma. Fallen stomas can be corrected by surgery.

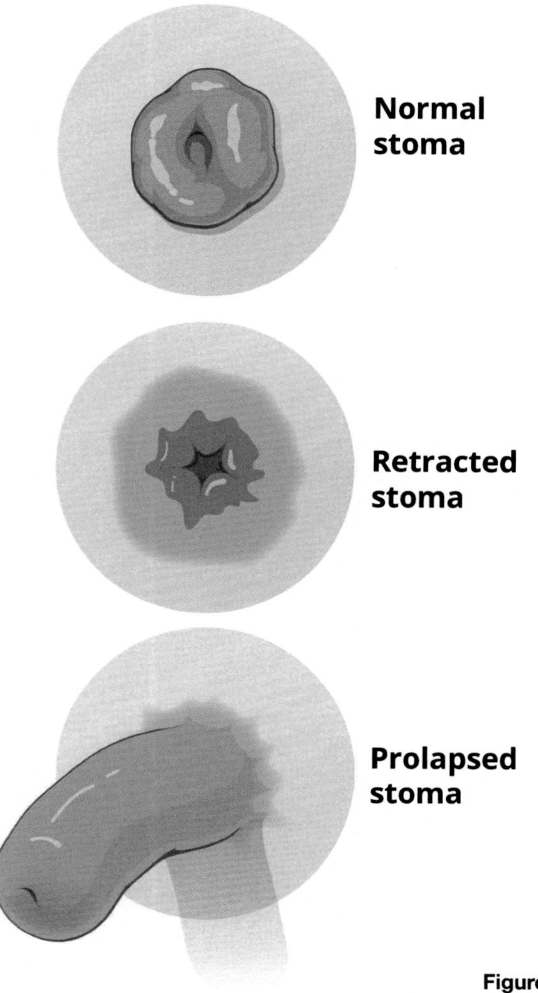

Figure 17.8
The different types of stoma hernias

Chapter 18

My "Neo" Bladder

Urinary Diversion

Patients who have a cystectomy no longer have a bladder, so they lose the natural reservoir for their urine. Your surgeon will develop a urinary diversion (alternate route to handle your urine), which your body will continue to produce.

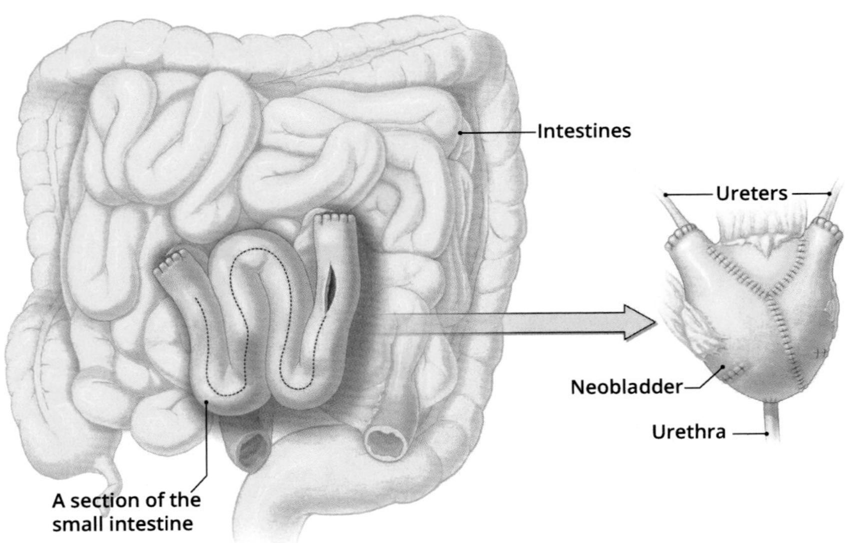

Neobladder

What is a neobladder?
A neobladder (from the Latin word "neo", meaning "new") is a pouch constructed from a segment of your small intestine. It will fulfill the same role as a normal bladder and will drain from your own urethra. This means that there is no stoma and no bag.

Receiving a successful neobladder means you will urinate similarly to the way you did before your surgery. Some patients need to use a catheter to empty their neobladder, but most do not.

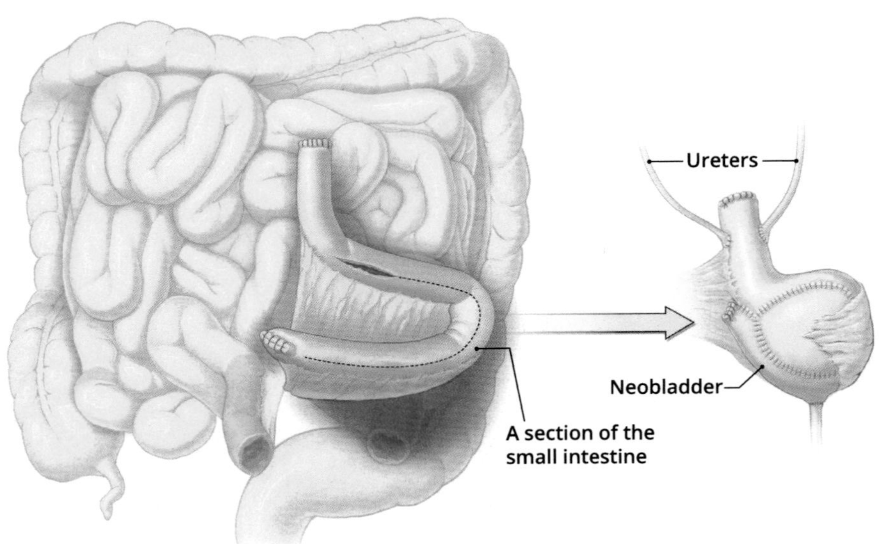

Figure 18.1
Hautmann and Studer techniques for a neobladder

Am I a candidate for a neobladder?
About 15-20% of patients who undergo cystectomy in our practice are candidates for neobladders. The most important factor is whether the urethra and kidney function can be preserved. The neobladder's best attribute is that it uses the patient's own urethra to drain the urine. Unfortunately, many bladder cancers invade the urethra and it must be removed. Without a urethra, there is no benefit to a neobladder and a pouch that you empty by catheter may be constructed instead.

How is a neobladder made?

After removing the diseased bladder, the surgeon separates a bowel segment (at least 45 cm) from the far end of the small intestine. Your surgeon fashions this length of intestine into a pouch (neobladder) within the abdomen where your bladder had been. This pouch is then attached to the ureters on top and the urethra below. Where the bowel segment is removed, the two free ends are joined to put the bowel back together.

The neobladder can be fashioned in several ways. The Hautmann and Studer techniques are two of the most common (illustrated in Figure 18.1). Your surgeon will determine which way will work best to create a low pressure, high-volume reservoir that functions as much as possible like normal bladder, without damaging the kidneys.

What is the difference between a neobladder and a normal bladder?

Our normal urinary bladder is a very specialized organ. It easily expands in size and volume due to its elasticity, and its muscular layer contracts strongly to drain urine quickly. The neobladder is constructed from the small intestine and unlike the bladder, the small intestine secretes mucus and has an outer layer that is neither as elastic nor as muscular as the natural bladder.

This leads to a few major concerns:

1. The mucus can become thick and cause obstructions.

2. The neobladder does not contract to empty itself, and it does not have an internal sphincter muscle to hold in the urine at rest. For these reasons, patients must learn different strategies to control their urine, and it will take time to develop continence again.

3. The neobladder does not connect to the same nerves as the bladder and does not send the same signals to the brain when it begins to stretch. Therefore, the familiar sensation of needing to urinate will not occur. Instead, the sensation has been described as a "fullness," similar to what you feel following a large meal.

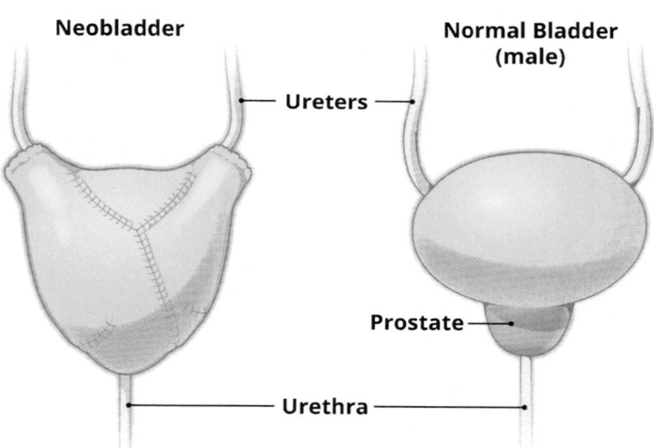

Figure 18.2
Comparing neobladder and normal bladder anatomy

How do I manage these concerns?

Your neobladder will need to be irrigated several times per day with sterile water or saline using a catheter. This prevents mucus from clogging the stents and the catheter.

You must drink enough water so that (a) the mucus stays thin and (b) enough urine is produced to flush it out. Drinking eight glasses of water per day is recommended.

Continuing to irrigate your neobladder after the catheter is removed is important. Once you regain control of your pelvic floor muscles, (see Chapter 22 on pelvic floor exercises) you will have more control over holding your urine. Until then, you may need to wear pads. Emptying the neobladder requires external pressure because the neo-bladder cannot produce the pressure itself. This maneuver is more similar to defecating than normal urination. Until you are proficient in fully emptying your neo-bladder, you will need to use a catheter. In some patients, this becomes necessary long term.

Even without the normal fullness sensation, you must urinate regularly with a neobladder. The neobladder will slowly develop more volume and elasticity over time, but it cannot handle being stretched the way a normal bladder can. Patients will need to urinate and drain the neobladder at least every two to four hours during the day and twice during the night.

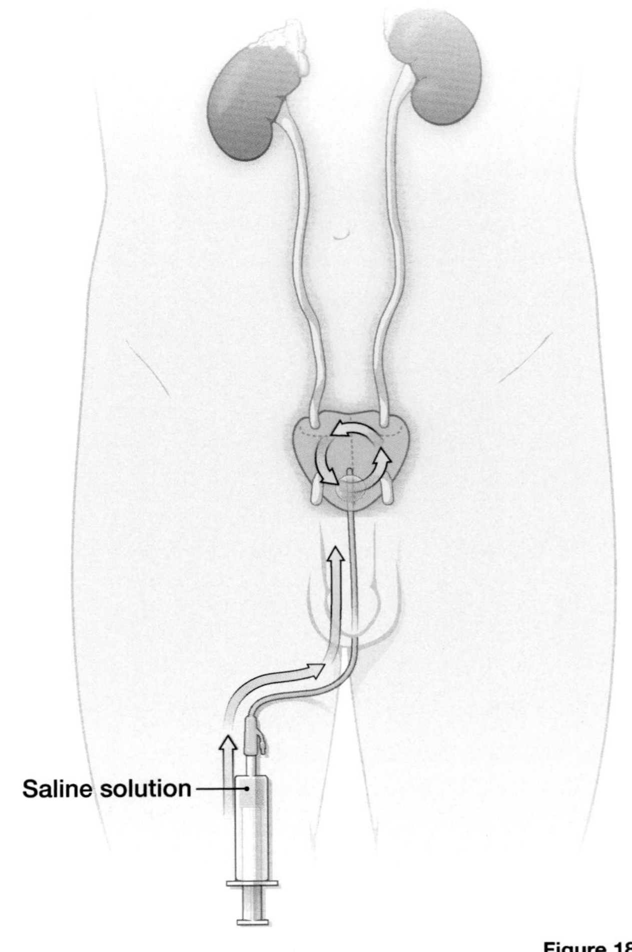

Figure 18.3
Neobladder being irrigated with saline solution

What complications might I expect with a neobladder?

Cystectomy with the creation of a neobladder is major surgery and involves a total remodeling of your pelvic anatomy. The urinary diversion itself, rather than the cystectomy, causes most complications.

Figure 18.4
Chart comparing normal bladder and neobladder functions

	Normal bladder	Neobladder
External Configuration	Normal	Similar to normal, performed by refashioning of the bowel
Continence Mechanism	Internal and external sphincters	External sphincter only
Voiding Mechanism	Contraction of bladder wall (once the brain gets signal fullness)	Straining and Crede* method. Some patients may require using a catheter.

Voiding Sensation	Sense of fullness and urge to void	Absent, because the nerves responsible for such sensations are removed with surgery. Patients may feel some abdominal fullness or discomfort (as eating a big meal).
Bladder Volume	Once adult volume is reached, usually remains the same	Distends with time
Junction with Ureters	Prevents reflux of urine from the bladder to the ureter	Usually allows reflux to the ureters which may lead to risk of kidney infections
Pressure Inside the Bladder	Low pressure is maintained to protect the kidneys from damage	Pressure is relatively high, then decreases as the neobladder distends with time
Mucus Production	None	Yes, since neobladder is made of intestine, which normally secrets mucus. However, mucus production decreases with time. Irrigation is required to avoid mucus buildup.
Absorption of Urine Constituents	None	Yes, as the normal function of the intestine is to absorb different ions and compounds, absorption occurs and may lead to some metabolic imbalances. Therefore, it cannot be created in patients with impaired kidney functions.

** Crede is method by which urine is manually expressed by applying pressure with hands on lower abdomen.*

Chapter 19

My Hospital Stay

MY HOSPITAL STAY

The day of your surgery, you will be cared for in three different rooms – the prep room, the operating room, and a recovery room. Here is what to expect from each room.

The Prep Room

In this room you will be given medications through an intravenous (IV) to help you to relax and sleep before going into the operating room (OR). An anesthesiologist or anesthesia technician will monitor you while you are under this medication. A blood pressure cuff will be wrapped around your arm so that your heart rate can be monitored. You, your bed and some of the equipment will be brought to the operating room.

The Operating Room

Here, all the staff will wear uniforms, masks, gloves and caps to protect you from infection. You will be moved onto the operating table and your arms and legs will be secured gently for the procedure.

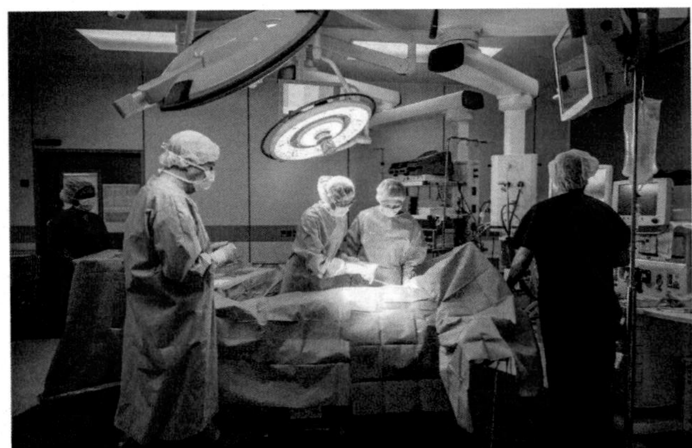

JohnnyGreig/iStock

The Recovery Room

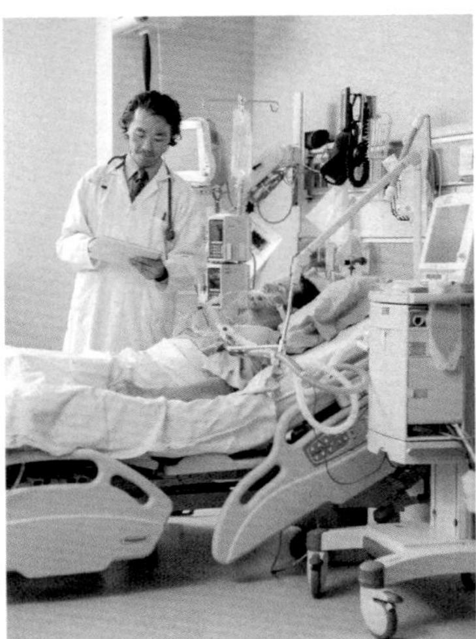

Tyler Olson/Shutterstock, Inc

After the surgery is completed, you will be moved to a recovery room. Here you will be watched closely and cared for until the effects of your anesthesia have worn off. When you wake up, you may find that your vision is blurry. This is caused by the medicine used to protect your eyes during surgery. The blurriness will go away in a short time. You may not remember much for up to 24 hours after surgery.

You may also have:

- Extra oxygen delivered through a thin tube passed into your nose (called a nasal canula).
- A catheter to drain urine from your body into a bag (known as a Foley catheter).
- A drain to remove excess fluid from your belly from the surgery (known as a Jackson-Pratt or Blake drain).
- Special stockings that squeeze your legs to help with your legs intermittent circulation and prevent clot formation. (These are known as sequential compression devices).
- An IV will remain in your hand or arm. Let your nurse know if there is any redness, or swelling or if you feel any irritation at your IV site.
- Dressing over the surgery area.

- A nasogastric tube, which goes through your nose to your stomach. This allows your body to rest and heal and helps to prevent bowel complications as you recover.

The Hospital Room

After you have recovered from the anesthesia (which can take a few hours), you will be moved to your hospital room for the rest of your hospital stay.

More about the Jackson-Pratt drain

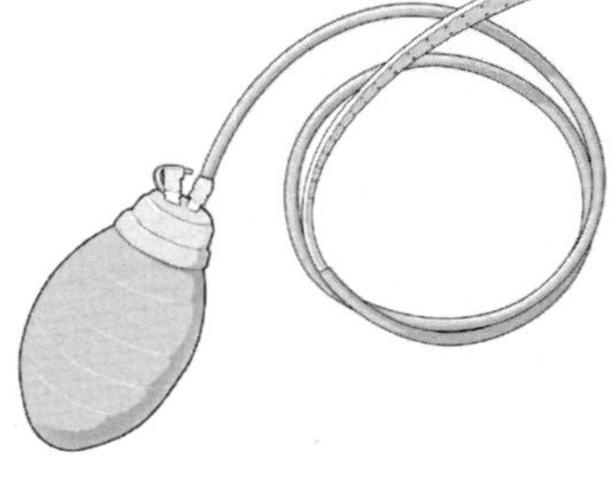

This drain is a suction device in which the drain itself is inside the body. It is made of Teflon material with multiple draining holes. It is connected to a clear plastic tube that is stitched to your skin where it leaves your body. The tubing connects to a bulb reservoir. When squeezed empty, the bulb applies constant suction to the drain, pulling fluid out of your body. The drain is removed when the excess fluid diminishes or stops.

How to care for the drain

You may be discharged with the drain in place. To care for your drain, you will need the following supplies:

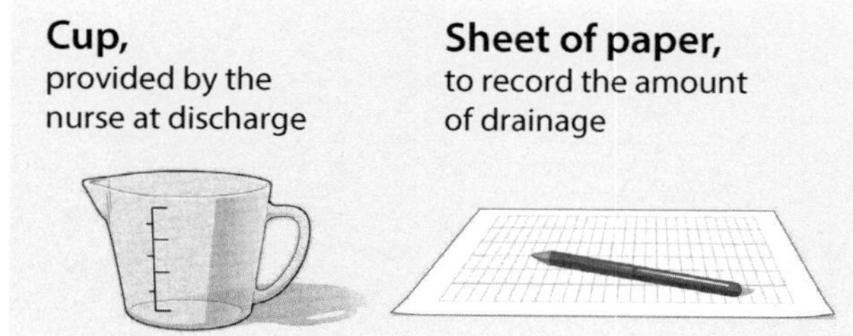

Figure 19.1
Supplies

Steps for Cleaning Your Drain

Wash your hands thoroughly with soap and water before and after you clean the drain. You will need to empty your drain twice a day. Discard the drainage once in the morning and once in the evening, at the same time each day, and record how much fluid was removed.

Figure 19.2
Steps for draining the Jackson-Pratt drain

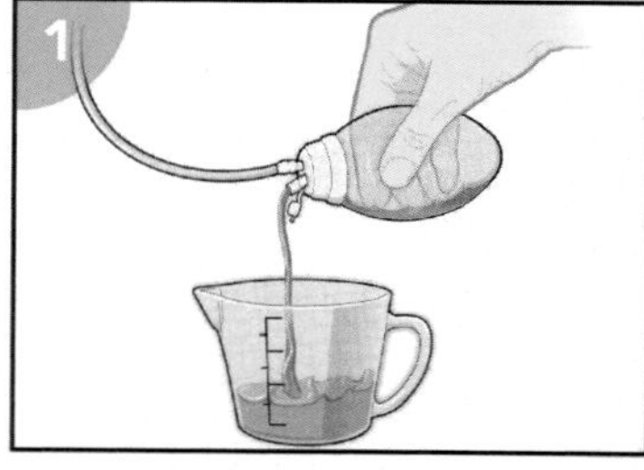

Pull the stopper out of the drainage bottle and empty the drainage fluid into the measuring cup.

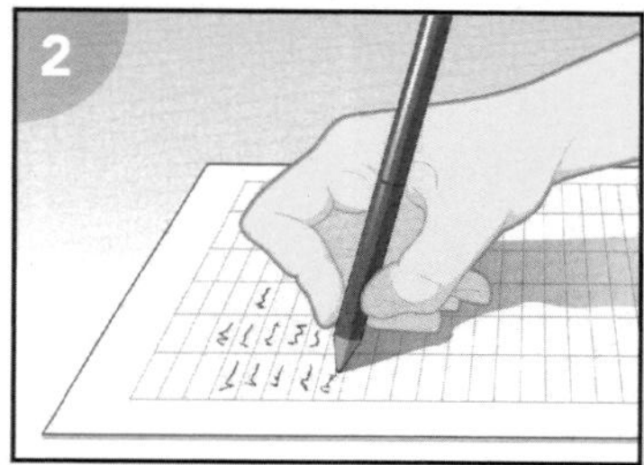

Record the amount of drainage fluid in your sheet.

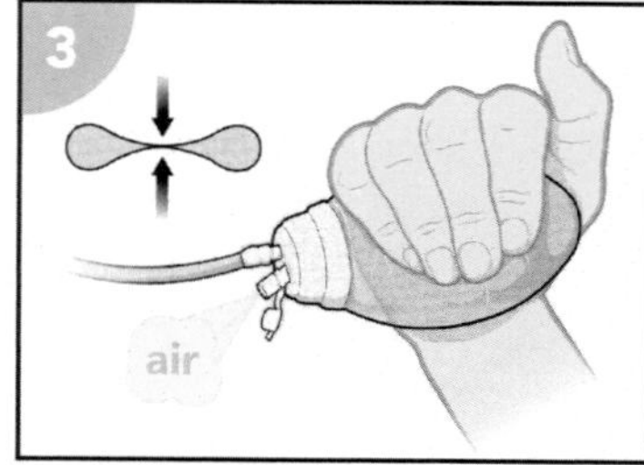

Squeeze the drain in the palm of your hand until the inside walls of the drain touch.

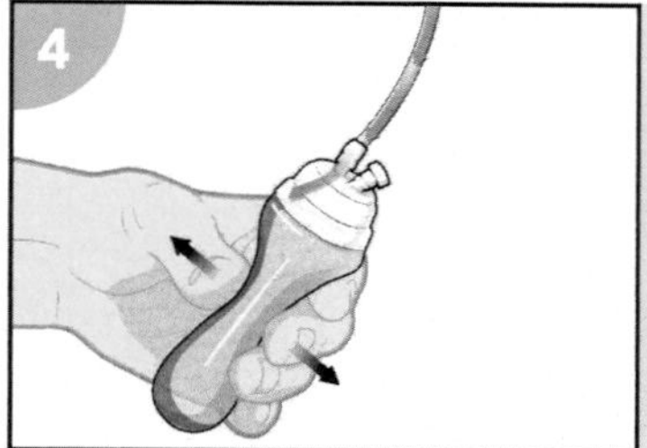

Replace the plug. Slowly release the grip to re-establish suction.

Continued on next page

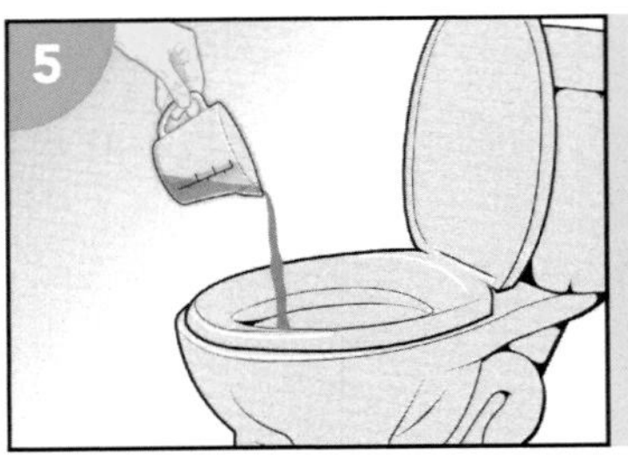

Dispose of the drainage fluid in a toilet or rinse it down a sink.

The drain should remain somewhat flat. If it is not flat, the suction is not working. Unplug the stopper and repeat step #3.

Pain Management with a PCA Pump

Patient-controlled analgesia (PCA) is a pain management method that allows you to control the amount of pain medication you receive. PCA uses a pump to deliver pain medications, either intravenously (with a needle inserted into your vein), or as an epidural (with a catheter inserted into the space around your spinal cord). A nurse will set the pump's controls so it will automatically deliver pain medication in a specific dose as prescribed by your doctor.

Depending on what your doctor prescribes, your pain medication may be delivered continuously or only when you press the button to activate the pump. For both methods, the pump is set to wait several minutes before another dose can be released, so you do not need to worry about overdosing on your medication.

Figure 19.3
The PCA pump

Use the pump to reduce your pain and keep it at a level you can tolerate. Do not wait until your pain gets worse to give yourself pain medication. If you wait too long, it may be difficult to get comfortable again and more pain medicine will be required.

Friends and family should not activate the pump for you, thinking they are helping to relieve your pain. You could end up receiving more medication than you actually need, which may increase the side effects. Remember, only you know how you feel, so you are the best judge of when you need the pain medication. Certain types of pain medications may aid in bowel recovery without affecting pain control. You should discuss these oral and non-narcotic options with your physician.

Getting Discharged

Your doctor will determine when you are able to go home. When you are discharged, a member of your healthcare team will give you the following:

1. Written discharge instructions (Do not hesitate to ask for additional help or information.)
2. Prescription for pain medicine (You may also receive stool softener medication.)
3. An appointment for your first follow-up visit.

Caring for yourself at home

Each day after your surgery you will feel better. These general instructions will help your recovery:

1. Keep your wound clean and change the dressing as instructed.
2. Increase your activity each day to prevent clot formation. Walk outdoors and use the stairs.
3. When sitting, prop your feet on a stool or sit on a recliner to keep your feet elevated and prevent swelling in your legs. If swelling occurs, lie in bed and rest your feet on a pillow higher than your head.
4. Do not resume driving until your doctor gives the okay and you are off narcotic medications.
5. Do not lift anything heavier than five pounds (e.g., a six-pack of soda) without permission from your doctor.
6. Continue to use your incentive spirometer breathing exercises each hour while you are awake.
7. Resume your usual diet as tolerated. Small, frequent meals help you tolerate food better.
8. To prevent constipation, eat foods higher in fiber, such as whole-grain breads and cereals and unpeeled, raw fruits and vegetables.
9. Drink five to six glasses of water or liquids every day.

Figure 19.4
Temporary stents

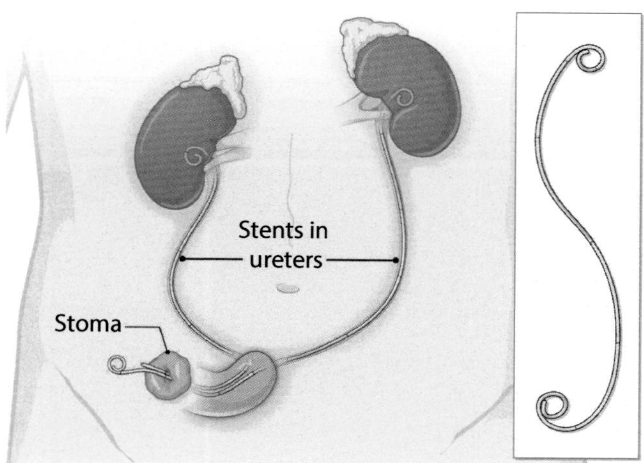

Ureteral stents are left in place for healing. The stents will either fall out on their own, or are removed by your health provider within two weeks of surgery. The stents are curled on both ends for them to stay in place. Sometimes the surgeon will cut the stoma end of the stent. Do not panic if they fall out. Please make sure you can identify the curls at the ends of the removed stent, which ensures that the complete stent is out (see Figure 19.4). Sometimes it is easier to take a picture to show your physician before discarding the stent.

Chapter 20

Possible Complications

POSSIBLE COMPLICATIONS

Radical cystectomy is a major surgery and even with the best surgeons, complications may occur. Complications can be classified as general (such as those that may follow any major surgery) or procedure-specific (such as those that may occur after radical cystectomy and urinary diversion.) Diversion-related complications may differ according to the type and technique of your diversion.

Complications can also be classified according to their severity. Physicians commonly use the Clavien-Dindo system, which classifies complications according to how they are managed and their consequences.

- **0** - no complication
- **I and II** - requires fluids or medications
- **III** - requires intervention
- **IV** - results in a disability
- **V** - death

The following charts summarize the complications that may occur after radical cystectomy and urinary diversion.

General

- Heart problems
- Collapsed lung due to accumulated secretions obstructing the airways
- Aspiration (when stomach contents are regurgitated and reach the airways)

Vascular

- Deep vein thrombosis, or blood clots in the deep veins of the legs. Clots may detach, circulate and block other vessels. They are particularly–worrisome if they reach the lungs, a condition known as pulmonary embolism (PE), which can be fatal.

Gastrointestinal

- Loss of bowel function.
- Stress ulcers of the small bowel or the stomach, may cause bleeding. Patients with peptic ulcers and those who use medications such as non-steroidal anti-inflammatory drugs are at higher risk.
- Diarrhea

Genitourinary

- Urinary tract obstruction
- Kidney failure
- Fistula (abnormal opening between structures, such as the vagina and the neobladder)

Infections

- Urinary tract infection
- Sepsis (Infection reaching the bloodstream)
- Wound infection
- Lung infection

Figure 20.1
Complications

Figure 20.2
Complications

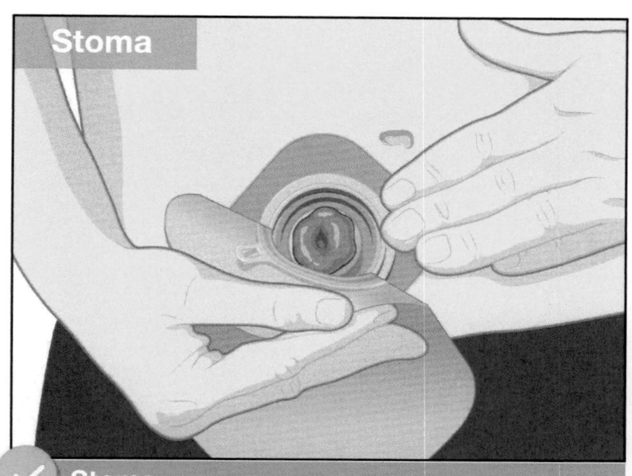

Stoma

- Stenosis (narrowing of the urostoma)
- Necrosis (darkening and tissue death of the part of the bowel forming the stoma).
- Skin rash

Abdominal Wall

- Parastomal hernia (protrusion of abdominal contents besides the urostomy).
- Incisional hernia (protrusion of abdominal contents through the incision).
- Wound failure. This problem may occur at the level of the muscles and fascia (causing hernia), or at the skin (causing burst abdomen).

Quality of Life

- Emotional impact, incontinence, and erectile dysfunction.

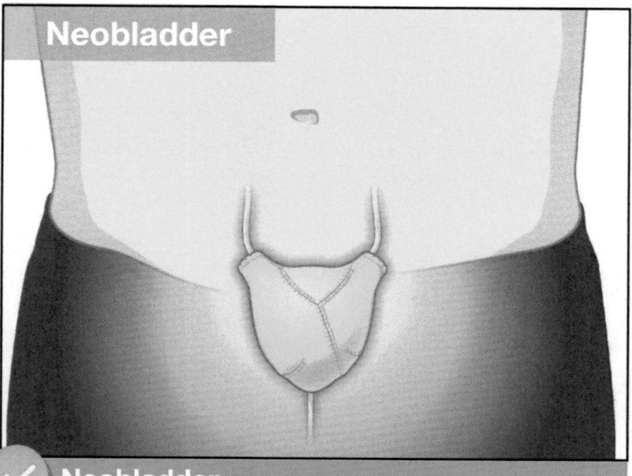

Neobladder

- Voiding problems (inability to void or involuntary escape of urine.)
- Rupture (very rare)

Procedure

- Leakage (Urine escapes through the suture lines. It may appear in the drain or accumulate inside the belly).
- Strictures: a narrowing of the ureters or urethra at the junction with the neobladder.

Metabolic

- Dehydration
- Electrolyte imbalance of certain substances in the blood, such as potassium, chloride and salt.
- Vitamin B_{12} deficiency

Continued on next page

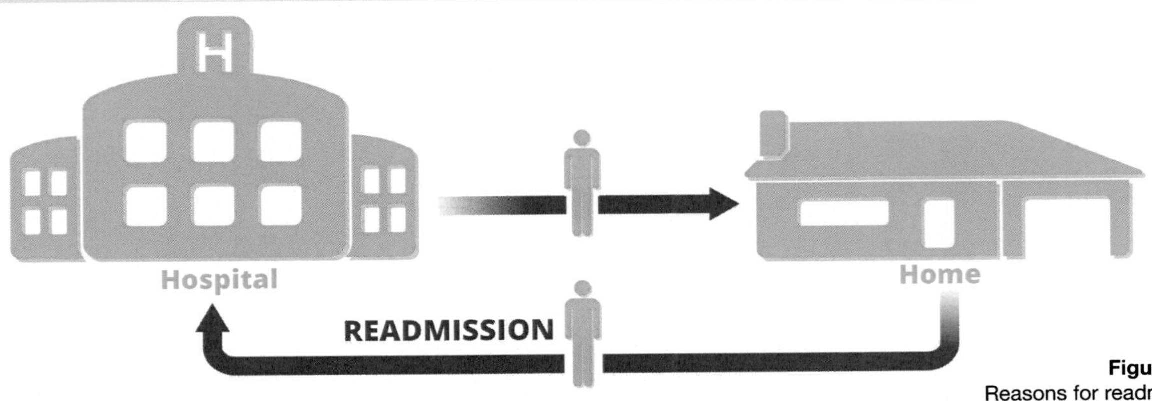

Figure 20.3
Reasons for readmission

Reason for Readmission

- Kidney infection
- Sepsis (infection reaching the bloodstream)
- Loss of bowel function due to paralytic Ileus and small bowel obstruction
- Ureteric stricture (narrowing at the junction between the ureters and the bowel forming the conduit or the reservoir)
- Deep vein thrombosis (DVT) or blood clots
- Respiratory complications (infections or lung collapse)
- Pelvic abscess (Infection at the surgery site, with pus)
- Dehydration
- Kidney failure and electrolyte disturbance
- Diarrhea
- Wound complications (Infection or wound failure)
- Leakage
- Fistula
- Heart attack
- Hypoglycemia (low levels of blood sugar)
- Others unrelated, such as inflamed appendix

Sometimes complications do not respond to medications or conservative measures. In those cases surgery may be required to fix the problem. The table below summarizes the main causes of reoperations following cystectomy. These procedures can be performed a few days after surgery, or months or even years later. A reoperation may be performed with minimally invasive techniques, (robot assistance), or open procedures.

Reason for Reoperation

- Bleeding
- Bowel injury during surgery
- Drainage of infection or abscess
- Compartment syndrome
- Revision of uretero-ileal strictures (narrowing)
- Fistula repair
- Hernia repair
- Bowel obstruction failing conservative management
- Kidney stones
- Revision of conduit e.g. due to stomal stenosis

Chapter 21

Unblocking the Urine

UNBLOCKING THE URINE

Urine may be blocked as a result of the healing process and as fibrous tissue (scar) forms, or less commonly, due to cancer recurrence. You may have no symptoms at all, or may experience flank pain (upper back, right below your ribs), fever or symptoms associated with kidney dysfunction (such as fatigue, anorexia, reduced urine output, nausea and vomiting).

If your urine is blocked, you may need a procedure called ureteroscopy. A ureteroscope a small, thin tube with a light and camera on the end. It is passed through the urethra and into the bladder. From the bladder, the scope is passed through a hole called the ureteral orifice that connects the ureters to the bladder.

This procedure can find various urinary tract problems, including kidney stones narrowing, and bladder tumors. Doctors can pass tiny specialized instruments through the ureteroscope to take a biopsy, treat kidney stones or remove a tumor. This is performed once the kidneys are unblocked.

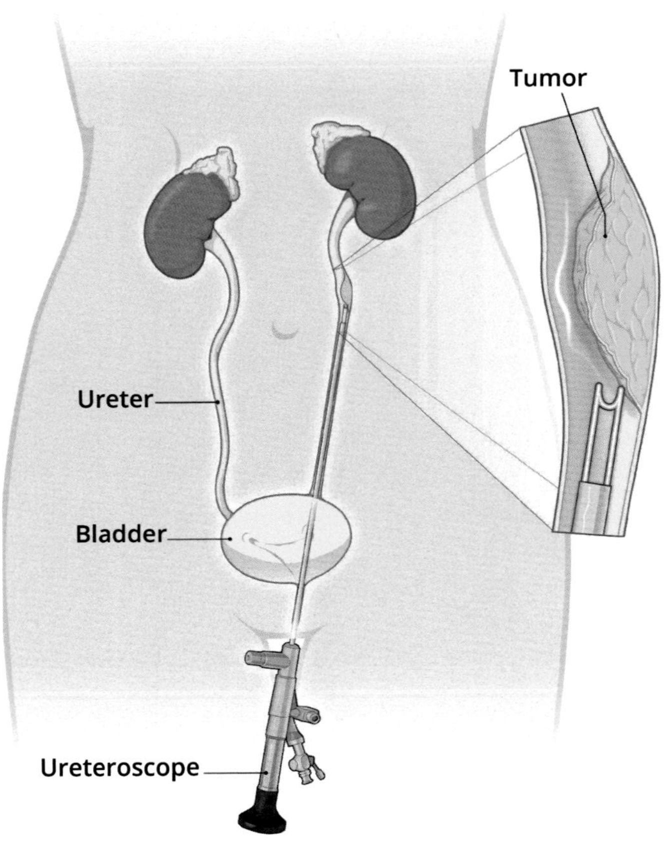

Figure 21.1
A flexible ureteroscope with a laser beam can shine through the fiber, breaking the tumor into smaller pieces that can then pass out of the body in the urine.

Types of Ureteroscopes

Currently–two types of scopes are used for ureteroscopy, flexible or semi-rigid–and each has advantages and disadvantages.

Flexible

Flexible ureteroscopes are used to safely negotiate the angles of the ureter. They can also access the entire upper urinary system in over 90% of patients.

Semi-rigid

Semi-rigid ureteroscopes are used only in the lower ureter because they are not long enough or flexible enough to reach the upper ureter or the kidney. However, they give doctors a better view and allow access to more instruments.

Why Would I Need a Ureteroscopy?

- **Surveillance:** To monitor any known conditions or tumors

- **Remove a tumor or growth:** Your doctor may use a pencil-like laser that emits an electrical current to cut tissue and stops bleeding.
- **Take a biopsy:** This is the best way to diagnose cancer in the ureters and pelvis of the kidney.

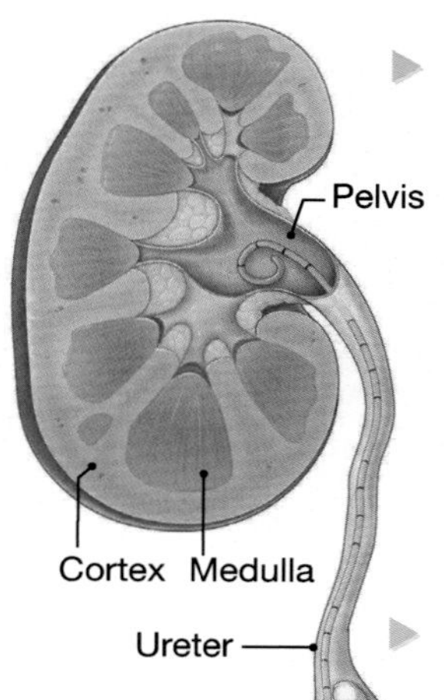

Figure 21.2
Ureteral stent inserted to relieve ureteral obstruction (cancer, stricture) and provide drainage.

- **Treat kidney stones:** Tiny mechanical devices (i.e. lasers) passed through the ureteroscope can break up stones and remove them.

Other Ways to Unblock Urine

- **Stent:** A ureteral stent is a thin tube placed into the ureter to prevent or treat urine obstruction from the kidney. Doctors may also insert the stent during surgery to allow the ureters to heal after suturing them to the bowel, or after surgery, if the ureters are strictured (narrowed).
- **Ureteral Dilation:** This procedure is commonly attempted to treat ureteral strictures (narrowing). Thin rods of increasing diameters are inserted through the ureter to widen the ureter without causing further injury.
- **Nephrostomy:** A nephrostomy creates a urinary diversion through an unnatural opening in the skin. This temporary solution provides urinary drainage for patients with blockage. It stays in the body only until a stent can be placed as a more permanent fix (typically within three weeks). If the urine is not redirected by nephrostomy, pressure builds up in the urinary system and the kidneys are damaged. Nephrostomy also provides your doctor access to the upper urinary tract for various endoscopic procedures.

How It's Done

A doctor makes an incision in your skin and inserts a tube into the kidney with the narrowed ureter. Urine leaves the kidney through the tube and into a collection bag outside the body rather than through the bladder.

What You Should Know

- The nephrostomy tube may be uncomfortable. It takes some getting used to.
- The tube attachments, bandages, skin barriers, and bolsters must be changed every seven days.
- The tube itself must be changed every two to three months by a doctor.

With a nephrostomy tube, you face a high risk of infection. Follow these instructions carefully to help avoid an infection:

1. Change bandages, skin barriers, and attachment devices as directed.
2. Wipe the connecting ends of the drainage bag with alcohol or iodine before you reconnect the bag to the tube.
3. Keep the tube taped to your skin and connected to a drainage bag placed below kidney level. This helps prevent urine from backing up into your kidneys.
4. A small drainage bag strapped to your leg allows you to move around more easily. Use a larger drainage bag at night and when napping to help prevent urine from leaking from the opening where the tube enters your skin.
5. Check the catheter to ensure it is in place after changing clothes or other activities. Place the tubing over your thigh rather than under it when sitting down. Be sure that nothing pulls on the nephrostomy tube as you move.
6. Change positions if you see little or no urine in your drainage bag. Check to see if the urine tube is twisted or bent. Be sure that you are not sitting or lying on the tube. If there are no kinks and there is little or no urine in the drainage bag, tell your caregiver and let your doctors know.

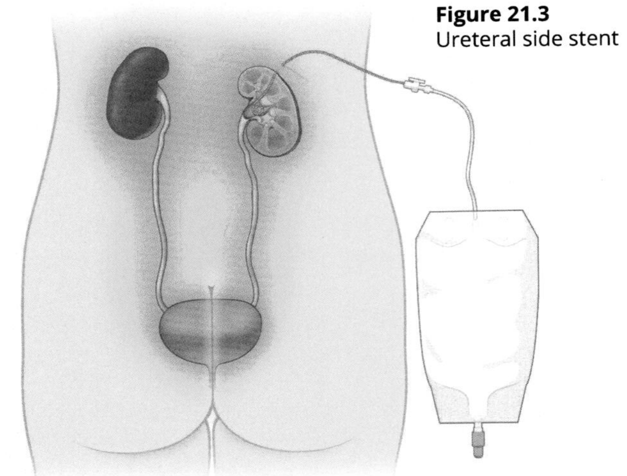

Figure 21.3
Ureteral side stent

7. Flush out the tube as directed. Do this if you think the tube is blocked. If the output from the tube is diminished, or takes longer than usual, it might be out of place.
8. Keep the site dry when you shower by taping a piece of clear adhesive plastic over the dressing. Do not take tub baths.

Seek Urgent Care If:

- The nephrostomy tube comes out completely.
- There is blood, pus, or a bad smell coming from the place where the tube enters your skin.
- Urine is leaking around the tube 10 days after the tube was placed.
- You have fever (>101.5°F), chills, or shivering.

Chapter 22

Postoperative Urinary Control

POSTOPERATIVE URINARY CONTROL

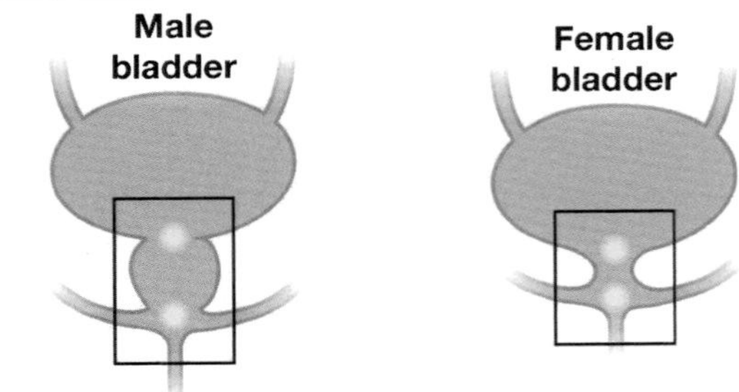

What Is Pelvic Floor Rehabilitation?

Pelvic floor rehabilitation is physical therapy that can help you control the pelvic floor muscles around the lower end of your (new) neobladder.

After bladder removal surgery, your neobladder does not have the support your original bladder had, and this makes it more difficult to hold urine. Pelvic floor rehabilitation will help you strengthen your pelvic floor muscles to better control urination.

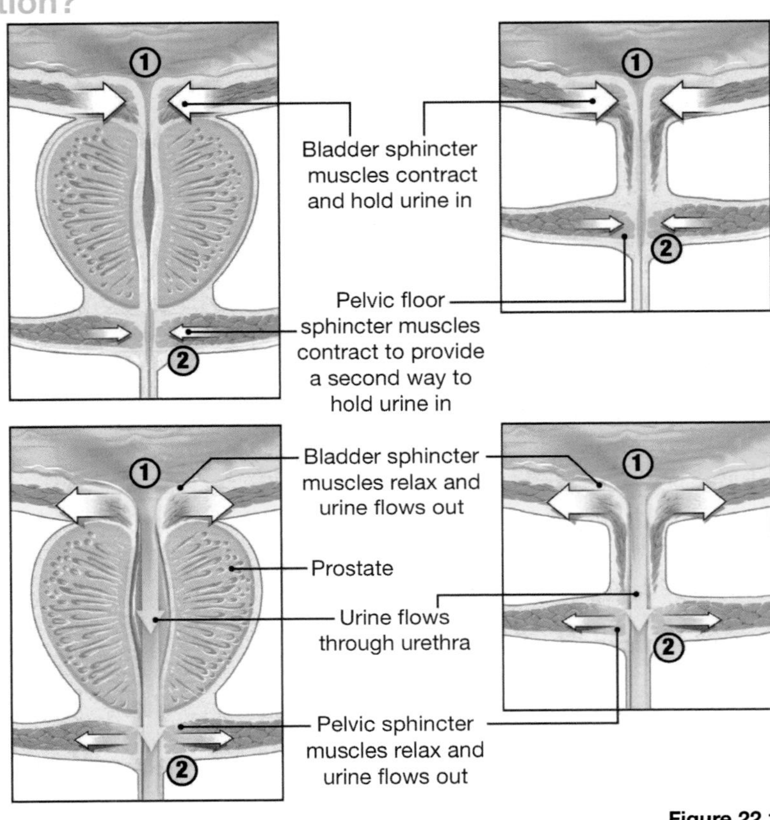

Figure 22.1
The two sphincters in men and women that control urination.

How Will My Body Change After Surgery?

Before bladder removal surgery:

- Your urine flows from your kidneys, down through two ureters and fills your bladder.
- A sphincter is a tight band of muscles that closes to hold urine and opens to allow urine to pass from your body.
- Your body naturally has two sphincters to control urination: external (voluntary) and internal (involuntary).
- In men, the internal sphincter is located between the bladder and prostate, and the external sphincter is located between the prostate and pelvic floor.
- In women, the internal sphincter is located between the bladder and the external sphincter.
- When you urinate, both sphincters relax to allow urine to flow from your bladder into your urethra and out of your body.

After bladder removal surgery:

- If you are a man, bladder removal surgery removes your bladder, prostate, the urethra that runs through your prostate (in men), and one of your two sphincters.

- After all these are removed, your neobladder will have to get used to all the changes.

How Will Urination Change After Surgery?

1. After your surgery, you may have to empty your bladder more often.
2. The shape of your neobladder and where it is positioned in your body will differ from your natural bladder.
3. The feeling you get when your bladder needs to be emptied will change. It will feel similar to stomach fullness, such as after eating a full meal.
4. It will take some time until you can recognize these new feelings in your body.
5. You may need to wear an underwear liner and use pelvic floor exercises while you learn to recognize these new feelings.

Continued on next page

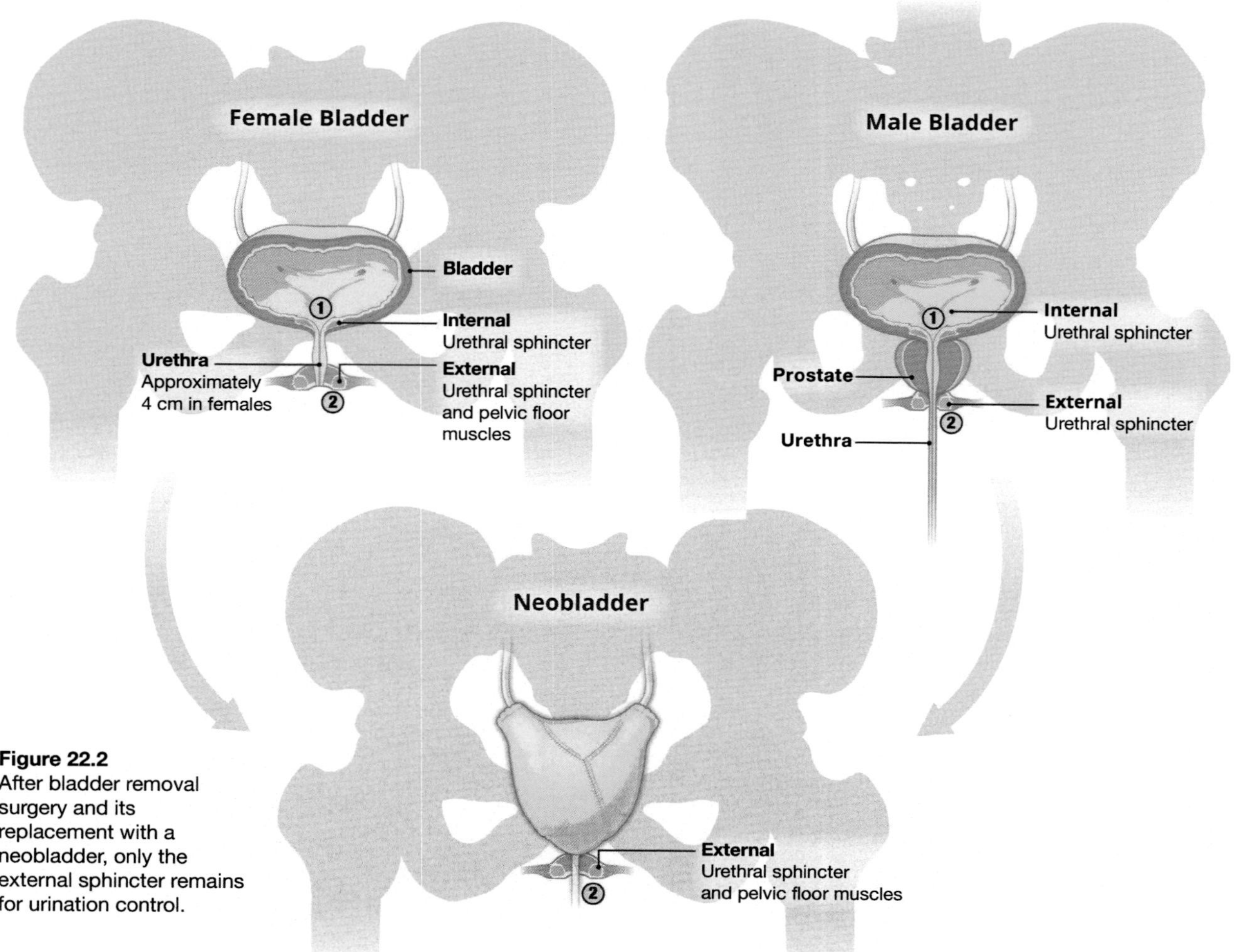

Figure 22.2
After bladder removal surgery and its replacement with a neobladder, only the external sphincter remains for urination control.

6. Pelvic floor exercises will help you recognize the feeling and prevent leakage.
7. Pelvic floor exercises will strengthen the remaining sphincter to help you regain control.

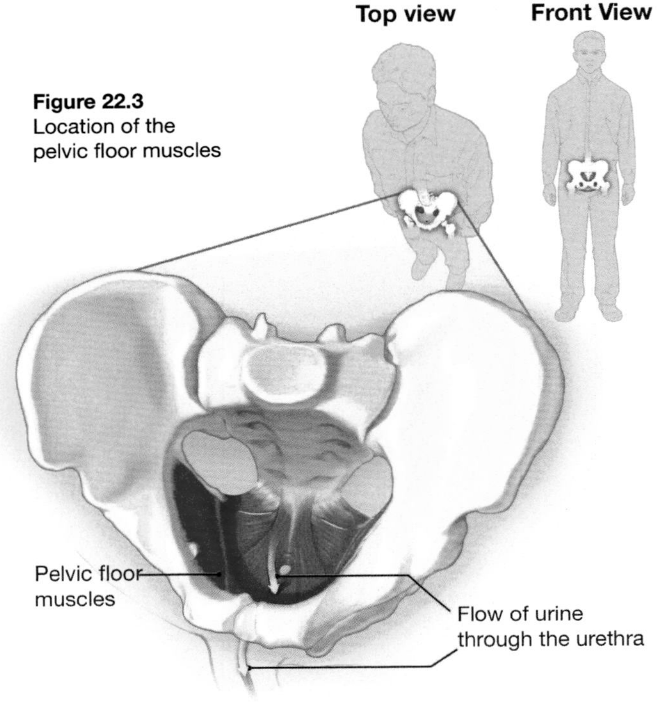

Figure 22.3
Location of the pelvic floor muscles

Why Exercise the Pelvic Floor?

After surgery: getting back on track

Doing pelvic rehabilitation on a regular basis and following dietary guidelines will help you adjust faster to the changes in your body and become more comfortable after surgery.

Improving urine control

Pelvic floor contraction exercises activate the muscles involved in urination and can help you improve urinary control. You don't have to set aside a special time or place to do these exercises. You can do them anywhere, anytime.

Try doing them while:

- Watching TV
- Sitting in the car at a stoplight
- Sitting at work
- Standing in the checkout line at the grocery store

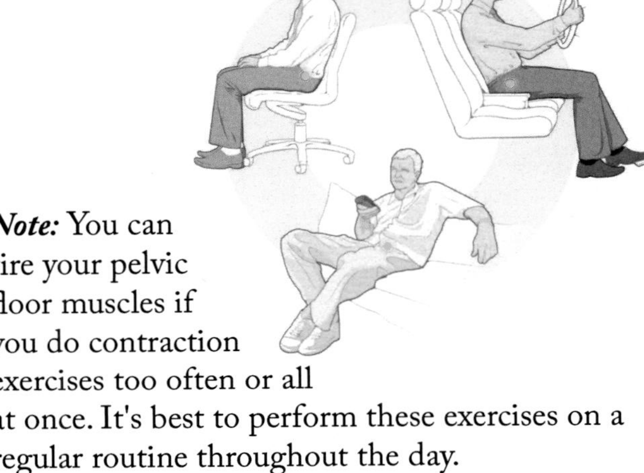

Note: You can tire your pelvic floor muscles if you do contraction exercises too often or all at once. It's best to perform these exercises on a regular routine throughout the day.

Steps for Locating Your Pelvic Floor (In Men)

The following exercises can help you locate your pelvic floor. Do the exercises until you are familiar with the tightening sensation between your legs. Your pelvic floor is in the area where you feel this tightening.

1. Gently squeeze the ring of muscles around your rectum (as if you were trying to avoid passing gas or stop a bowel movement).
2. While you are urinating, tighten your muscles to stop the flow of urine. (Do not do this all the time, or you may develop a habit of not emptying your neobladder completely.)

3. Stand in front of the mirror naked and look at your penis.

4. Without moving the rest of your body, try to make your penis twitch or move up and down.

Figure 22.4
Penile twitch - a method of observing if the pelvic floor muscle exercises are performed correctly

Penile twitch test

The pelvic floor can be located by tightening the perineum, the tissue between your scrotum or vulva and anus. By gently applying pressure to your perineum and tightening your pelvic floor, your perineum will move away from contact. A physical therapist or nurse can help you locate the pelvic floor muscles by palpating the perineum. This method can then be used yourself at home.

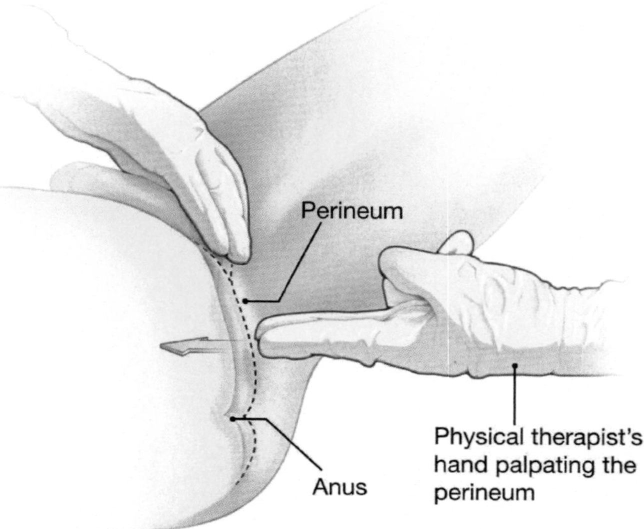

Figure 22.5
The perineum moves away from contact as the pelvic floor muscles contract

Now that you know where your pelvic muscles are, you can quickly activate them by squeezing and then relaxing to achieve the tightening sensation you felt in the exercises above.

Pelvic Floor Workouts

Exercise #1:
The one-second hold

00:01

1. Empty your bladder and relax.
2. Tighten your pelvic floor muscles and hold for one second. (You should feel the tightening sensation).
3. Relax the pelvic floor completely for 1 second. (Keep in mind that there is no quick "on/off" switch.)
4. Repeat Steps 2 and 3 (above) between 10 and 20 times.
5. Repeat this exercise as often as you can throughout the day, in different positions (sitting, standing, and lying down).

Exercise #2:
The 10-second hold

1. Empty your bladder and relax.
2. Tighten your pelvic floor muscles and hold for 10 seconds.
3. Slowly relax the pelvic floor muscles completely for 10 seconds.
4. Repeat Steps 2 and 3 (above) between 10 and 20 times.
5. Repeat the exercise five times throughout the day.

At first you may not be able to squeeze the muscle for the full 10 seconds. The more you practice, the easier it will become. If your muscles get tired after six or eight repetitions, stop until you feel relaxed again, and then continue. This exercise will build your endurance.

Doing It Right

Learning to do pelvic rehabilitation correctly from the very beginning – being careful to work just the pelvic muscles – can make a big difference in how well you can control your bladder.

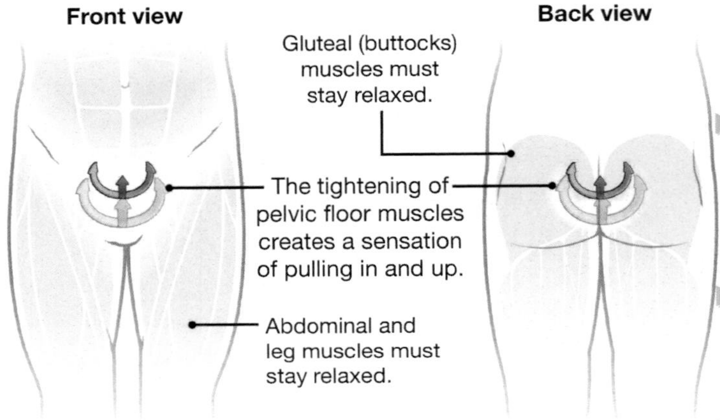

Figure 22.6
Relaxed muscles of the abdomen, legs, and buttocks are a good indicator that the pelvic floor exercises are done correctly.

Tips for exercising correctly:

- Do not use the muscles in your stomach, legs, or buttocks. To avoid using your stomach muscles, place a hand on your stomach while you squeeze your pelvic floor. If you feel your abdomen move, you are using the wrong muscles.
- Do not hold your breath, because that will put pressure on your abdomen.
- It is easier to prevent leaks than to stop them after they begin. Remember to tighten your pelvic floor before you sneeze or cough, or while you are changing position.

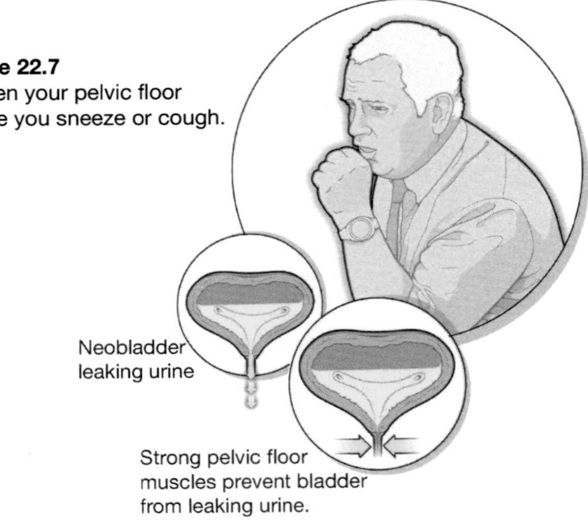

Figure 22.7
Tighten your pelvic floor before you sneeze or cough.

- Continue your exercises regularly even if your symptoms increase at first. You will improve over time. (Tighten evenly throughout a change in positions.)
- You should see some improvement in your symptoms after just a few weeks of exercise.
- Make your pelvic floor contraction routine a part of your daily life. As with any exercise, you will have to continue to work your muscles in order to maintain their strength.

Other Options for Urine Control

Slings (both men and women)
If pelvic floor exercises fail to improve urine control, surgical options may help.

If your urine control problems are not severe, you can gain full control over your bladder using a male sling. In this procedure, surgeons make one small cut near your perineum and place a mesh sling. The sling puts pressure on your urethra, which holds your urine in, to help keep it from leaking.

Figure 22.7
InVance® Male Sling system

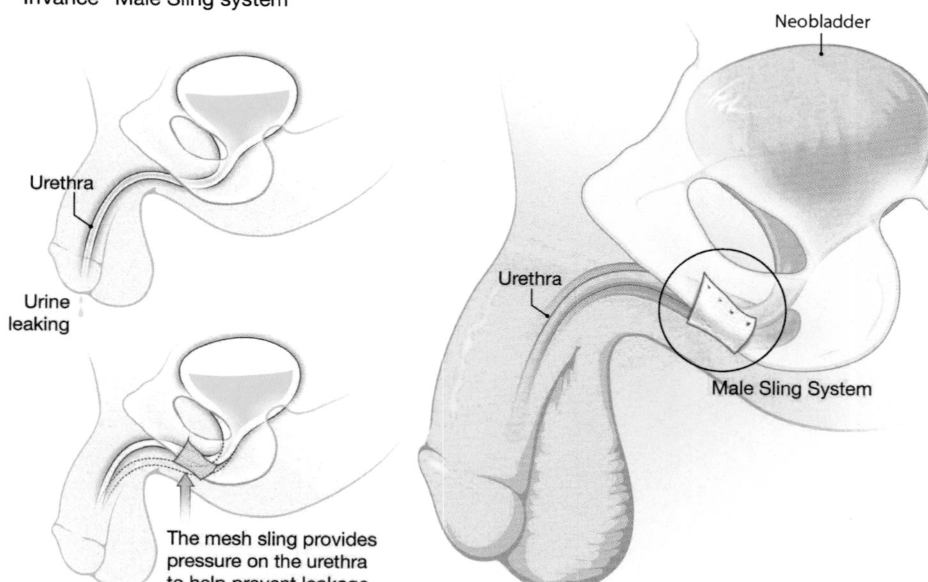

When the cuff closes, it inflates a pressure-regulating balloon near your bladder, which keeps the urine from leaking.

To urinate, all you need to do is press a button on the control stick placed in your scrotum. The cuff starts to depressurize, and urine will begin to flow. Then press the button one more time when you are done.

If you think there is still some urine left, just press the button again to empty your bladder.

Some medical conditions, such as osteomyelitis and severe osteoporosis, can make this treatment harmful for you. Be sure to talk to your medical team first.

Pressurized urinary control system (only in men)

If your urine control problem is far more severe and difficult to manage, the urinary control system can help you gain control of your urine.

Normally, your sphincter controls the flow of urine by opening and closing your urethra. But with a neobladder, your sphincter loses the ability to open and close the urethra, and you lose control of your urine.

The urinary control system works by surgically inserting a cuff that acts the way your sphincter did.

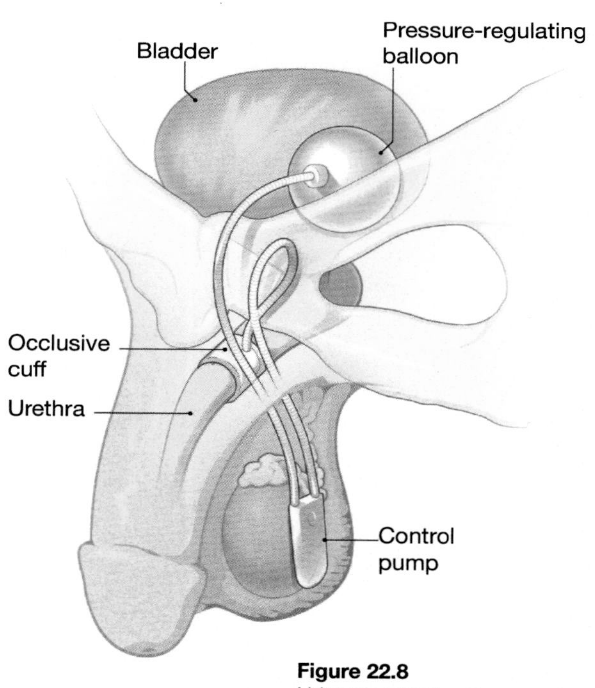

Figure 22.8
Urinary control system

Chapter 23

Coping With Sexual Side Effects

COPING WITH SEXUAL SIDE EFFECTS OF TREATMENT

Depending on type of treatment, you may experience some effects on your sexual function. This may range from a temporary change in your libido (sex drive) during chemotherapy to longer-term changes. Coping with sexual changes after treatment can be very difficult, because you may have lasting physical effects of your illness, and this can affect the closeness and intimacy you feel with a partner, too.

It will be important for you to speak openly about these concerns with your medical provider, because a number of treatment options are available. If you find it difficult to discuss this topic with your partner, you may want to seek the assistance of a counselor in your treatment center. Counselors are comfortable discussing these symptoms and routinely help patients and couples find ways to re-engage sexually after treatment.

What Side Effects Can I Expect After Surgery?

For women, side effects from chemotherapy may be short-term or long-term, depending on treatment type and duration. Short-term effects may include a decrease in libido. Long-term effects, such as early menopause, may be experienced, such as difficulty with arousal, difficulty achieving orgasm, or painful intercourse. Painful intercourse may also occur with vaginal dryness from radiation therapy, or vaginal shortening or tightening from surgery. Some women struggle with body image concerns related to changes in their body structure and function.

For men, treatment with surgery and/or radiation therapy may contribute to erectile issues or dry orgasm. Dry orgasm occurs when a man reaches sexual climax but does not ejaculate semen. This is typically not a problem with sexual pleasure, but can be if a man is hoping to father children. Men may also struggle with body image concerns after radiation and surgery, and in coping emotionally with changes in sexual function.

What Options Can Help With These Issues?

A number of potential interventions can help with sexual side effects. For women experiencing vaginal shortening and tightening, dilators are often used with good success. Lubricants or estrogen treatment may relieve vaginal dryness, and menopause symptoms may be managed with hormones.

FOR WOMEN

Figure 23.1

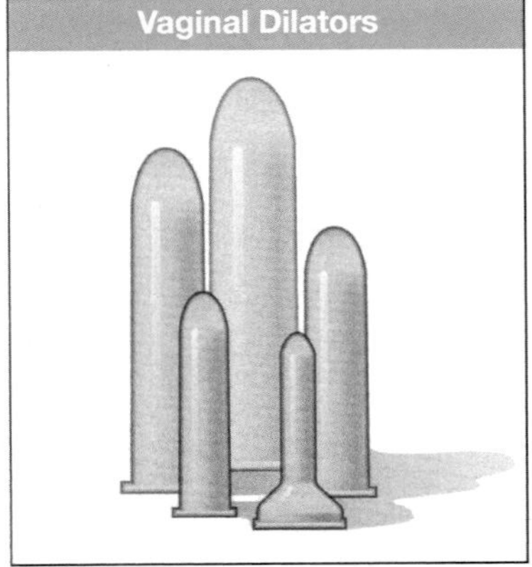

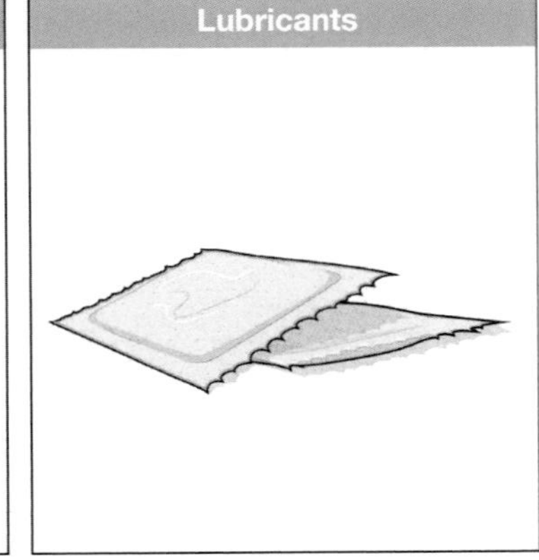

For men experiencing erectile issues, a number of options are available, including medication, intraurethral pellet therapy, a vacuum erection device, or a penile prosthesis. Your medical team can tell you more about these options.

FOR MEN

Figure 23.2

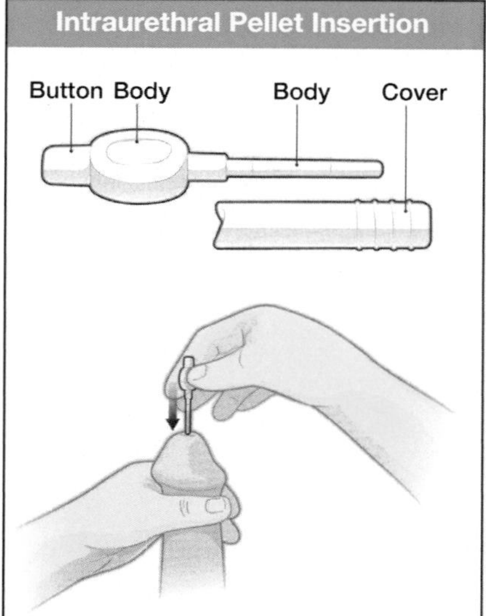

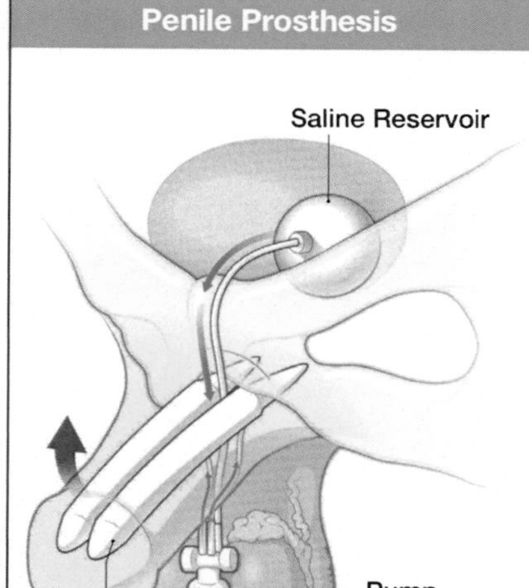

For anyone experiencing sexual side effects from treatment, a number of support resources are available to you. Ask your treatment team about educational materials and respected websites for more information on treatment options.

What Can I Expect From a Visit with a Sex Therapist?

Many people find it uncomfortable to discuss their sex life, whether with their partner or their medical team. Sex therapists are clinicians trained in working with patients and couples experiencing difficulties with intimacy and sexual satisfaction.

While your sex life may need to change a little after cancer treatment to accommodate changes in your function, it is expected that you can return to a satisfying level of intimacy again.

A visit will likely include discussion of the current problems along with what has worked well in the past. While this discussion may initially feel awkward or uncomfortable, it will be beneficial to talk openly about an area of your life that is important to you. The therapist will likely give you tasks or "homework" to work on between sessions to help you and your partner discover what can work well for you. A few sessions with a therapist may allow you to return to a level of closeness and intimacy that you both find fulfilling.

Chapter 24

Chemotherapy, Radiation and Other Treatment Options

CHEMOTHERAPY, RADIATION AND OTHER OPTIONS

The right treatment for you will depend on many factors, such as your disease characteristics, invasiveness or stage and your overall health status. Chemotherapy and radiation therapy are treatments that target cancer cells and are commonly used methods to treat side effects and limit the tumor's spread. They can be given along with surgery or instead of surgery if an operation is not feasible for you and you have symptoms.

Chemotherapy

Chemotherapy drugs are delivered in various ways and will depend on your disease stage, drug characteristics, toxicity, and your preference.

More than 100 chemotherapy drugs are used to treat cancer, and your physician will choose your specific drugs and drug combination, based on your individual needs.

Bladder-Preserving Combined Modality Therapy (CMT)

This treatment is an option for patients who are not eligible for surgery due to other medical problems. CMT is an alternative to surgery if you wish to refuse surgery and keep your bladder. Your physician will recommend CMT for you depending on your disease histology, stage, kidney function and health status. CMT consists of three treatments: extensive TURBT, to maximally remove the entire tumor in a safe manner, radiotherapy, and chemotherapy.

Although CMT seems promising in selected patients, it is not yet recommended as standard first line of treatment for muscle-invasive bladder cancer.

Systemic Chemotherapy if Not Eligible for Surgery

Systemic chemotherapy refers to drugs taken either orally or directly infused into the bloodstream. The drugs are not confined to the bladder but circulate throughout the body. Systemic chemotherapy provides a stronger effect in terms of survival and disease control but may come with greater side effects.

Adjuvant Chemotherapy

If you did not receive neoadjuvant chemotherapy (before surgery), you may be evaluated after surgery to determine whether you should receive it now. This is known as "adjuvant chemotherapy."

The National Comprehensive Cancer Network (NCCN) recommendations state that patients with muscle-invasive bladder cancer can benefit from adjuvant chemotherapy that includes a platinum-based drug (e.g. Cisplatin).

If your final pathology reveals that your cancer is not confined to the bladder, or if the margins of the removed tissue contain bladder cancer, chemotherapy may delay recurrence, although overall survival benefit might be modest.

Because different drug combinations have never been compared in a randomized clinical trial, no agreement has been reached on the ideal combination of chemotherapies. However, research shows that the ideal regimen should include at least two drugs, with one drug containing a platinum component (such as cisplatin and gemcitabine).

Side Effects of Chemotherapy

Because chemotherapy drugs travel through your whole body, other cells may be affected by the drugs, too, especially rapidly dividing cells such as those of the intestinal lining, bone marrow and hair follicles.

Chemotherapy side effects depend on the drug's dosage and the length of exposure. Common side effects include fatigue, nausea, vomiting, loss of appetite, diarrhea, hair loss, dry skin, bleeding, bruising, and a higher risk of infections. Side effects are usually temporary and are relieved shortly after finishing treatment. Medications may be given to help control and alleviate such symptoms as nausea, vomiting, or diarrhea.

More profound side effects may occur with treatments that last longer and may persist even after stopping the drugs. These may include nerve damage that can lead to abnormal sensations, hearing loss, or peripheral neuropathy, which causes pain, burning, itching, or loss of sensation. Other side effects include lung fibrosis, heart failure, or memory problems. Adriamycin may cause heart failure.

Radiation Therapy

Radiation therapy (or radiotherapy) uses high-energy waves to damage the cancer cell DNA and kill the cells. For many patients with advanced invasive bladder cancer and symptoms, radiotherapy may be an alternative option.

Radiation is generated outside the body from a large machine outside the body and directed toward the tumor. This is known as External Beam Radiation Therapy (EBRT). Different doses of radiation can be directed toward the tumor site. Radiation therapy can be used:

- Instead of surgery, as a bladder-preserving combined modality therapy (CMT) with TURBT and chemotherapy.
- To alleviate pain in patients whose cancer has spread to their bones.
- Local control of advanced bladder cancer (e.g., severe bleeding).

TURBT may cause side effects; fatigue, nausea, vomiting, diarrhea, dry skin, and irritative urinary symptoms such as burning, pain, or blood in the urine. (See Chapter 6 for more on TURBT.)

Most of these side effects are temporary and go away after treatment is complete. However, some patients may experience severe problems, such as inability to control urine (incontinence) or inflammation of the bladder, which causes pain and bleeding while passing urine (radiation cystitis).

Clinical Trials

Cancer researchers continually aim to develop better ways to treat cancer. Before any potential new drug or treatment can be used on patients, it must undergo years of intensive study in both the laboratory and clinical setting.

Clinical trails are the final stages of study before a new agent becomes an approved drug. Most clinical trials will test a new treatment by comparing it to the existing standard treatment. Every standard cancer treatment–and all drugs, for any medical condition–started out as studies in clinical trials.

Treatments in clinical trials can be either biological (living or naturally occurring substances), or artificial, man-made substances.

You must first give permission to join the trial if you want to receive these potential new drugs.

As a participant in a clinical trial, you may be asked to provide additional information about yourself. Doctors will conduct multiple tests (blood work, scans) to measure the effectiveness of the treatment.

You are never required to participate in a clinical trial. If you do enroll in a clinical trial, you can stop participating at any time. Clinical trials are experimental, which means there is a risk that the treatment will not work at all. However, all clinical trials in the United States must pass through an Institutional Review Board (IRB). The person in charge of the trial must prove to the IRB (based on laboratory research and science) that there is a good chance that the treatment will work.

Chapter 25

Survivorship: Life After Treatment

SURVIVORSHIP: LIFE AFTER TREATMENT

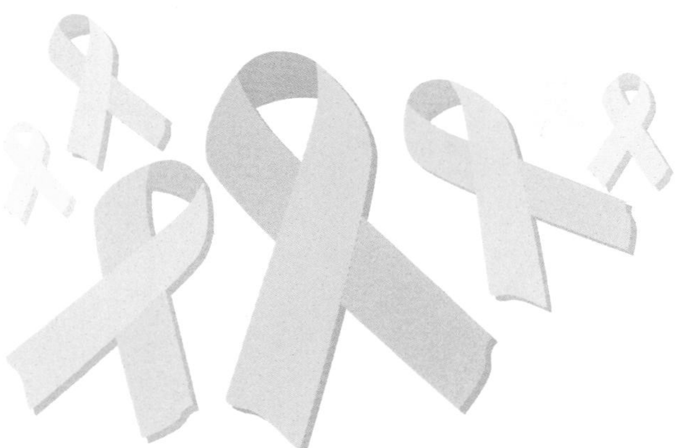

Completing treatment for bladder cancer can be both an exciting and stressful time. To be finished with active treatment and on the road to healing is a relief for most patients, but for many it also includes a transition to a number of new considerations. This transition from active treatment is often called "survivorship", and is now seen as a distinct phase of cancer treatment.

What Can I Expect as I Move into Survivorship?

A major area of concern for many patients is ongoing treatment-related symptoms. Symptoms such as fatigue or pain will likely subside the further you get from treatment. Other symptoms, however–such as sexual side effects or emotional concerns such as anxiety, fear or depression–may only now be coming to the surface. In addition, you may be returning to prior roles and responsibilities at work, with family, or caring for an elderly parent.

Many patients are distressed to find that the support that was present during treatment is now diminishing, at a time when they continue to feel fatigued and have mounting stress and responsibilities. If any of these issues persist after treatment ends, inform your medical team so they can connect you with a survivorship care program.

What Resources Will Be Useful?

Seek the assistance of your medical team to prepare you for what to expect after treatment ends. Ask for a referral to a therapist who can help you cope with the emotional impact of your cancer experience, stress associated with upcoming scans (called "scanxiety") or with depression. Many patients make this a time to re-prioritize how they would like to live their lives, and a counselor can be helpful in working through this.

A nutritionist may help you learn healthier eating habits, and a physical therapist can show you how to resume exercise. Engaging in healthy lifestyle habits such as not smoking, eating a healthy diet, and exercising regularly may not decrease your risk of developing a new or recurrent cancer, but those steps will help reduce the risk of further health problems.

Survivorship Care Plans

Many treatment centers provide patients with a summary of what to expect as treatment ends.

Your care plan should include:

- An outline of follow-up testing
- Future cancer screening exams
- Possible short- and long-term side effects of treatment–what to watch for, and when to notify your doctor

- Healthy lifestyle recommendations (including nutrition and exercise guidelines)

Since completing treatment, I am very concerned that my cancer will come back. What can I do?

Concern that your cancer may return is a very common and normal response after treatment. You may find it useful to speak with other cancer survivors, in a support group or one-on-one, to learn about their coping strategies. The American Cancer Society and Cancer websites have useful information on coping with fear of recurrence, along with a number of other survivorship concerns.

While it may feel that much is outside of your control when it comes to a cancer recurrence, try to focus on what is in your control: following your treatment plan, attending all follow-up appointments and testing visits, and maintaining a healthy lifestyle.

Many services are available to help you manage ongoing symptoms after treatment, including educational resources and websites, and services provided by your treatment center or community providers. Talk to your treatment team about how to receive the help you need to manage this new phase of life.

Chapter 26

If My Options Seem Limited

IF MY OPTIONS SEEM LIMITED

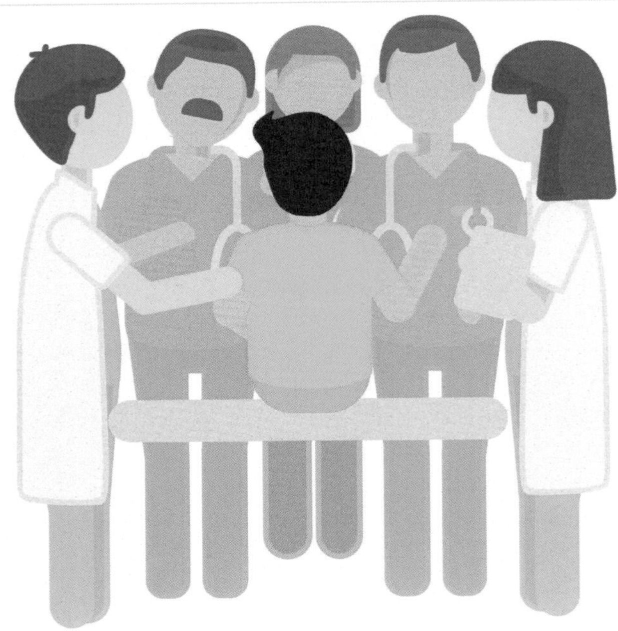

Despite your medical team's best efforts your cancer may still progress, and it can be a major source of physical, emotional and spiritual pain. Complications associated with cancer can lead to lifestyle changes that are overwhelming, and can adversely affect your social life. Fortunately, many services are available to help you cope.

Palliative Treatment

Palliative treatment is designed to improve your quality of life. Palliative care offers pain and symptom relief, emotional and spiritual support, and comfort to patients and their families.

Not to be confused with hospice or end-of-life care, palliative care can be utilized at any stage of an illness and at the same time treatment is given to try to cure the cancer. In advanced cancer, palliative treatment may help you live longer and more comfortably, even if you cannot be cured. For example, treatment may help reduce pain by shrinking a tumor, relieving pressure on nerves or surrounding tissues.

The palliative care team includes:

- Specialist doctors and nurses
- Social workers
- Pastoral care workers, such as pastors or chaplains
- Other health care professionals, such as dietitians, physiotherapists and counselors

Common Symptoms

1. **Pain**
   If you are in pain, it is vital that you inform your medical team. Pain, or fear of pain, can be very stressful. Some patients worry about side effects associated with pain medication. Controlling your pain is much easier if you use medication as soon as the pain starts. Sometimes pain control becomes harder and takes longer if you delay using appropriate pain relief.

2. **Loss of appetite**
   People in the advanced stages of illness often lose their appetite. This might be related to other symptoms such as pain, nausea or fatigue. Different body processes slow down with illness, making it more difficult to digest food or to make good use of it.

   Do not to force yourself to eat if you're not comfortable or hungry (although others might want to encourage your eating.) Keep up your fluid intake and nutrition requirements with liquid meals, water, tea or whatever else you prefer.

3 **Fatigue**
General weakness may result from anemia, malnourishment, or failure of the bone marrow to produce new cells. Discuss this with your palliative care team.

4 **Delirium**
With more advanced disease, patients may become confused at times. Usually this is a result of an underlying cause, such as fever, infection, medication side effects or cancers that have spread to the brain. Your palliative care team can help make the confusion less distressing for you and your loved ones.

5 **Emotional distress**
Understandably, you may experience some very strong emotions, such as sadness, depression, anger and anxiety. Pastoral care and psychosocial specialists can help you and your family with these challenges. Treatment can make you more comfortable, too.

6 **Other problems**
Malnourishment, lowered immunity and the cancer's spread to adjacent organs or distant sites can cause bowel problems, infections, breathing problems or difficulty with passing urine. Your team can offer you options.

Hospice Care

If your cancer spreads to other areas of your body and stops responding to treatment or cannot be safely removed, you should look for strategies to help you lead a comfortable life for as long as possible, rather than going through drastic and risky treatments that are unlikely to work.

This can be a very hard truth for you and your loved ones. With acceptance, however, psychologically comes internal peace that can lead to a much better quality of life. Hospice care is end-of-life care usually provided to patients expected to live six months or less. A team of healthcare professionals provides palliative care (pain and symptom control and emotional and spiritual support) in addition to other services.

Hospice programs also provide services to support a patient's family. Hospice patients are most often cared for wherever they feel most comfortable such as at home, an assisted-living facility, or a hospice care facility.

Hospice care can provide a sense of hope and fulfillment as you live out your last days in comfort. Hospice may help build a sense of happiness and satisfaction with life, improve relationships, and encourage optimism and hope.

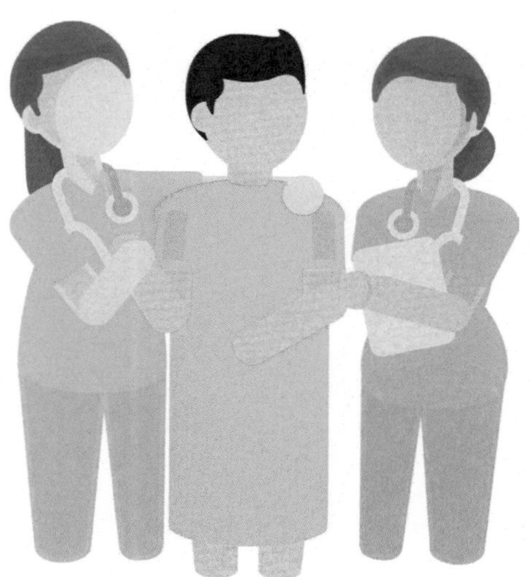

Radical Cystectomy Program at Roswell Park Cancer Institute

RADICAL CYSTECTOMY PROGRAM

Development of the Program

The Robot-Assisted Radical Cystectomy (RARC) Program at Roswell Park Cancer Institute was initiated in October 2005 when Dr. Khurshid A. Guru, MD, FABU, was appointed Director of Robotic Surgery. Dr. Guru completed his residency training in urological surgery and a robotic surgery fellowship at the Vattikuti Urology Institute, Henry Ford Health System in Detroit, MI. He also completed an international fellowship in urologic-oncology (2004) at the Urology and Nephrology Center at Mansoura University, Mansoura, Egypt.

Dr. Guru was one of the first fellowship-trained robotic surgeons and has more than 10,000 surgical console hours and more than 2,500 procedures to his credit. Dr. Guru performed one of the first robot-assisted radical cystectomies in New York state, and has worked on the development and evolution of oncologic safety and effectiveness of minimally invasive approaches to bladder cancer. Dr. Guru has performed live demonstrations of robotic surgery at international seminars in eleven countries.

Active collaboration with perioperative services, the robot-assisted surgery support team (nursing, operating room technicians and physician assistants) and the genitourinary pathology team lead to initiation of the RARC quality assurance program.

Goals of the Program

The short-term goal of the RARC program was to establish oncologic efficacy of radical surgery, optimize operative time and achieve adequacy of an extended pelvic lymph node dissection. An intracorporeal approach for urinary diversion (performed using the robot rather than through open incision, a common approach utilized by most surgeons at that time) began in 2009.

We also started a stringent multidisciplinary protocol in 2011 with our medical oncology department with strict neoadjuvant chemotherapy (NAC) consultation for all eligible patients. In 2012 we adopted a robot-assisted approach to all reoperation for diversion-related complications, which alleviated the associated morbidity of these challenging procedures. Finally, in 2015 we developed and popularized the robot-assisted intracorporeal technique for W-shaped neobladders, a bladder substitute urinary diversion that allows patients to live a near-normal life after this major surgery.

Outcomes

More than 525 cystectomies have been performed by our program since 2005. Measuring our outcomes over time demonstrated the impact of experience and interventions employed. Administration of NAC started initially at a low rate. Stringent incorporation of a multidisciplinary approach led to more than 90% of patients receiving consultation, and administration increased from 18% in 2009 to 40% in 2015. The overall utilization of chemotherapy prior to surgery is higher than the national average. Since 2009, almost all patients (>90% each year) have received intracorporeal (robot-assisted) urinary diversion. Despite this change, blood loss and operative times improved while complication rates remained stable. The positive soft-tissue surgical margins rate, which denotes adequate tumor resection, was only 7% and remained stable over a decade in spite of approximately half of our patients harboring a locally advanced disease.

Research

Dr. Guru has led his team to author and co-author more than 175 journal articles, abstracts, and book chapters. His efforts have been substantial in advancing the field of surgical education and the outcomes of RARC for bladder cancer. The research team, the Applied Technology Laboratory for Advanced Surgery (ATLAS), includes research fellows, biomedical and human factors engineers, database managers and coordinators, and a dedicated biostatistician in addition to interns and volunteers. Key research interests include:

1 Training and surgical education

Our program developed one of the first robotic surgical simulators, currently used in more than 20 institutions across the globe. Dr. Guru developed the first validated robotic surgery curriculum for safe transfer of surgical skills for future robotic surgeons. We developed and validated different scoring systems in collaboration with world-renowned experts. We have already published four scoring systems.

2 Outcomes research

We house the International Robotic Cystectomy Database (IRCC), the largest in the world. This is a multinational, multi-institutional database with 41 surgeons from 23 institutions in 14 countries. We developed and published a technique for intracorporeal W-neobladder to help popularize intracorporeal continent diversion. We participate in national and international collaborations and clinical trials to promote evidence-based strategic plans for patient management.

3 Quality control

We developed the Quality Cystectomy Score (QCS), which measures the quality of surgical performance independent of the patient and disease characteristics, allowing for consistent comparative effectiveness research among different bladder cancer programs. This score provides important information for patients insurance companies, and institutions to audit surgical performance. This work has been highlighted in the American Society of Clinical Oncology official newsletter.

4 Brain-computer interaction (Mind Maps project)

With advances in robot-assisted surgery, it became crucial to understand more about human brain and machine interaction, and how this affects learning, skill acquisition, mental and physical workload. We were the first to study the difference in cognitive function between experts and novices, as well as during different stages of surgery. We described the process of mentorship during robot-assisted surgery, and how this can help cognitive learning side-by-side with physical training.

5 Operating room environment for robot-assisted surgery (Techno-Fields project)

Introduction of robot-assisted surgery has been associated with changes in the operating room layout. The physical separation of the surgeon (at the console) from the patient and the rest of the team may affect communication and team dynamics in the operating room. We developed a methodology that captures different team activities during surgery, we mapped team dynamics as well as procedural interruptions, and reviewed methods that can optimize operating room performance and avoid adverse events. This research aims to provide an ideal work environment for the surgical team, minimizing adverse events, and improving patient safety.

6 Basic science

In collaboration with our basic science researchers, we are looking at the mechanism of local recurrence after bladder cancer, and the effect of pneumoperitoneum on peritoneal immune response against tumor cells. This work has been awarded "best poster presentation" by the American Urological Association (AUA 2016, San Diego). We are collaborating to develop bladder cancer organoids that can be used as models mimicking bladder cancer, and provide the ideal environment to investigate tumor behavior and response to different therapies.

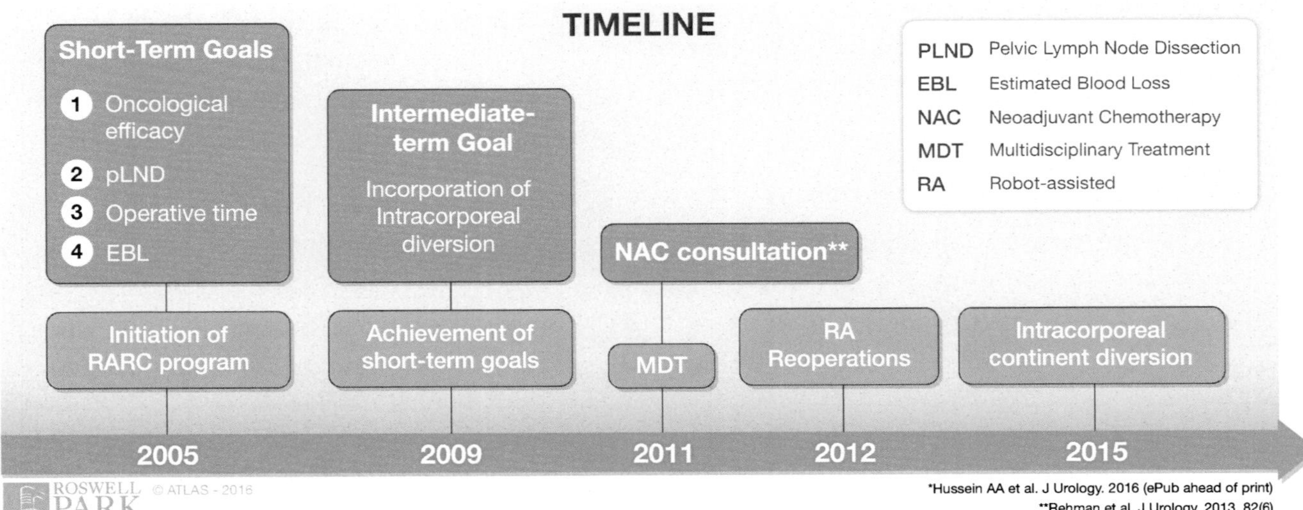

Glossary

A

Allergies - when your immune system reacts to a foreign substance.
Anemia - a condition in which your blood lacks enough healthy red blood cells
Anorexia - lacking the desire to eat
Artificial - man made substances

B

BCG - a weakened form of the bacterium that causes tuberculosis
Benadryl™ - used to treat sneezing, runny nose, watery eyes, itching, hives and rashes
Benign - describes tumors that cannot invade neighboring tissues or spread to other parts of the body
Biological - pertains to living organisms
Blood clots - a semi-solid mass of coagulated blood
Blood type - A, B, AB, and O. Each letter refers to a kind of antigen or proteins on the surface of red blood cells.
Bowel - the intestine

C

Catheter - a long tube that goes up your urethra into your bladder
Carcinoma - a common type of cancer cell that develops from epithelial cells, such as those in the bladder lining
Cervix - connects the vagina and the uterus
Chemotherapy - therapy that uses a chemical or combination of chemicals to kill cancer cells.
> **Adjuvant chemotherapy** - chemotherapy given after surgery.
> **Neoadjuvant chemotherapy** - chemotherapy given before surgery.

Clinical trial - clinical research in which promising new treatments are studied in human volunteers
Computerized Tomography (CT) scan - a way to produce cross-sectional images of the bones, blood vessels and soft tissues in your body by computer processing a series of x-ray images
Complication - a negative side effect
Coumadin - brand name for warfarin, a drug used to prevent blood clots
Cystectomy - a surgical operation to remove urinary bladder.

D

Defecating - passing stools; pooping
Dehydration - lack of enough fluids in your body, affects body's salt levels.

E

Endometrium - the mucous membrane lining the uterus, which thickens during the menstrual cycle in preparation for possible pregnancy
Embryo - an unborn offspring that occurs shortly after fertilization
Enoxaparin - generic name for Lovenox, an anti-coagulant used to prevent blood clots formation.

F

Fallopian tubes - women have two of these. They connect the uterus to the ovaries. When the egg is released from the ovary, it goes into the fallopian tube which carries the egg into the uterus.

Fetus - an unborn offspring of a mammal more than eight weeks after conception

G

Gastrointestinal - pertaining to the stomach
Genitals - external sex organs

H

Heart rate - number of beats your heart makes in a minute
Hernia - when an organ, or part of an organ, pushes through the wall of the cavity in which it normally resides
Hysterectomy - surgical removal of the uterus

I

Ileal conduit - formed using part of the small intestine, it's the easiest and most common urinary diversion urologists perform.
Ileum - part of small intestine
Immune system - made up of a network of cells, tissues, and organs that work together to defend the body against microorganisms
Incision - surgical cut made in the skin or flesh
Infection - invasion of body tissue by disease-causing agents
Intravesicular - delivered directly into the bladder

J

K

Kegel exercises - movements to build pelvic strength to help control urine.

L

Lymph nodes - small bean-shaped tissues in the lymphatic system, that serve important function for immunity and drainage.

M

MRI - magnetic resonance imaging a type scan used to examine different organs
Malignant - describes tumors that can invade neighboring tissues and spread to other parts of the body. Cells usually grow out of control.
Metastasis - when cancer spreads to other areas of the body far from the cancer's original site.
Mucus - a slippery substance secreted by mucous membranes

N

Nausea - upset stomach
Neobladder - "new bladder". It is a pouch constructed from a segment of the small intestine to replace the original bladder after removal.
Nerves - a bundle of fibers that transmit sensation impulses to the brain or spinal cord.
NSAIDS - non-steroidal anti-inflammatory drugs that relieve pain, i.e. aspirin, ibuprofen and naproxen

O

Orally - taken by mouth
Osteomyelitis - infection of the bone and the bone marrow
Osteoporosis - causes bones to be weak and brittle

Outpatient - a person who receives medical care without being admitted into a hospital.
Ovaries - about the size of a large grape. Females have two of these, one on each side of the uterus. They store and release eggs and secrete hormones called **estrogen** and **progesterone**.

P

Palliative care - provides relief from symptoms and stress in patients at any stage of treatment.
Papillary - long, finger-like tumors that stretch out from the bladder wall toward the center of the bladder
Pelvic floor - muscles around the opening of the bladder
Pelvic rehabilitation - physical therapy to strengthen the muscles around the bladder opening
Plavix - a brand name for clopidogel, medication that prevents platelets from sticking together and forming a clot
Pneumonia - a lung infection
Preoperative visit - a special medical appointment scheduled within a month before surgery
Prostatectomy - surgical removal of the prostate gland

Q

R

Radiation therapy - treating disease using x-rays or similar forms of radiation.
- **External radiation** - radio waves are beamed from outside the body to your tumors.
- **Internal radiation** - through a special procedure, the radioactive substance is placed directly onto your cancer.

Radical cystectomy - surgical removal of the bladder and some of the surrounding lymph nodes.

S

Self-catheterize - to place a urinary catheter yourself to empty the bladder
Seminal vesicles - pair of small tubular glands located in the pelvis behind the urinary bladder in men
Sepsis - a bacterial infection of the bloodstream.
Sperm - male reproductive cell
Spirometer - a special device that measures lung volume
Sphincter - ring of muscles located at the beginning of the urethra. The sphincter controls the flow of urine.
- **External sphincter** - a voluntary sphincter that you can control to urinate
- **Internal sphincter** - an involuntary sphincter that our body controls for us

Spine bone lesions - caused by nerve root compression
Small intestine - part of the intestine between the stomach and the large intestine.
Smallpox - an infectious disease caused by the variola virus
Stent - a small tube used to treat urinary obstruction of ureters
Sterile - free of bacteria
Stoma - opening through the skin near your belly button

T

Testicles - organs in men that produce sperm and the hormone testosterone
Tumor - any abnormal growth of cells, whether benign or malignant

Transurethral resection - a procedure to remove cancerous tissue from the bladder through the urethra using a scope
Tuberculosis - a serious infectious lung disease, caused by the bacterium mycobacterium tuberculosis

U

Uterus - also known as the womb. It is a pear-shaped organ located on top of the bladder and part of female reproductive system.
Urethra - a small tube that allows urine to travel from the bladder to outside your body.
Ureter - a tube like structure that carries urine form the kidney to the bladder
Urinary diversion - a way to reroute the path urine takes to exit the body. It is needed when the normal route is disrupted due to disease.
Urinary tract infection (UTI) - when bacteria affect any part of the urinary tract

V

Vaccine - a biological preparation that provides immunity to a particular disease; often contains a weakened agent of the disease.
Voiding log - chart of every time you urinate

W

X

Y

Z

References

Bibliography

Wilson TG, Guru K, Rosen RC, et al. Best practices in robot-assisted radical cystectomy and urinary reconstruction: recommendations of the Pasadena Consensus Panel. European Urology. 2015; 67(3):363-375.

Raza SJ, Wilson T, Peabody JO, et al. Long-term oncologic outcomes following robot-assisted radical cystectomy: results from the International Robotic Cystectomy Consortium. Eur Urol. 2015; 68(4):721-728.

Eisenberg MS, Boorjian SA, Cheville JC, et al. The SPARC score: a multifactorial outcome prediction model for patients undergoing radical cystectomy for bladder cancer. J Urol. 2013; 190(6):2005-2010.

Rehman S, Crane A, Din R, et al. Understanding avoidance, refusal, and abandonment of chemotherapy before and after cystectomy for bladder cancer. Urology. 2013; 82(6):1370-1375.

Poch MA, Raza J, Nyquist J, Guru KA. Tips and tricks to robot-assisted radical cystectomy and intracorporeal diversion. Curr Opin Urol. 2013; 23(1):65-71.

Azzouni FS, Din R, Rehman S, et al. The first 100 consecutive, robot-assisted, intracorporeal ileal conduits: evolution of technique and 90-day outcomes. Eur Urol. 2013; 63(4):637-643.

Abol-Enein H, Tilki D, Mosbah A, et al. Does the extent of lymphadenectomy in radical cystectomy for bladder cancer influence disease-free survival? A prospective single-center study. Eur Urol. 2011; 60(3):572-577.

Hussein AA, Dibaj S, Hinata N, et al. Development and validation of a quality assurance score for robot-assisted radical cystectomy: a 10-Year Analysis. Urology. 2016.

Hautmann RE, de Petriconi RC, Pfeiffer C, Volkmer BG. Radical cystectomy for urothelial carcinoma of the bladder without neoadjuvant or adjuvant therapy: long-term results in 1100 patients. Eur Urol. 2012; 61(5):1039-1047.

Stein JP, Lieskovsky G, Cote R, et al. Radical cystectomy in the treatment of invasive bladder cancer: long-term results in 1,054 patients. Journal of Clinical Oncology. 2001; 19(3):666-675.

Herr HW, Faulkner JR, Grossman HB, et al. Surgical factors influence bladder cancer outcomes: a cooperative group report. Journal of Clinical Oncology. 2004; 22(14):2781-2789.

Hinata N, Hussein AA, George S, et al. Impact of suboptimal neoadjuvant chemotherapy on peri-operative outcomes and survival after robot-assisted radical cystectomy: a multicentre multinational study. BJU Int. 2017; 119(4):605-611.

Hussein AA, Ghani KR, Peabody J, et al. Development and validation of an objective scoring tool for robot-assisted radical prostatectomy: prostatectomy assessment and competency evaluation. J Urol. 2016.

About ATLAS

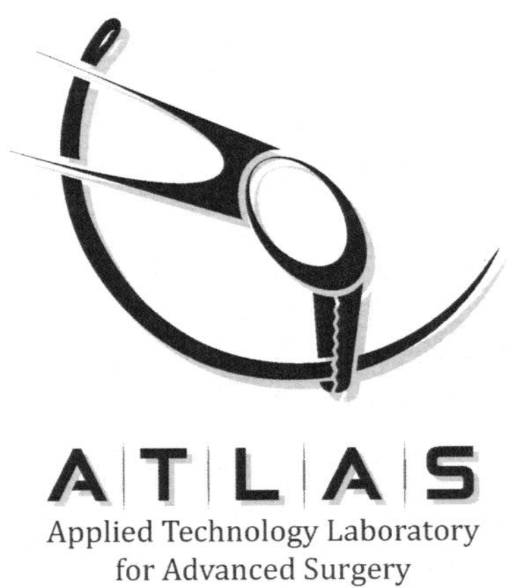

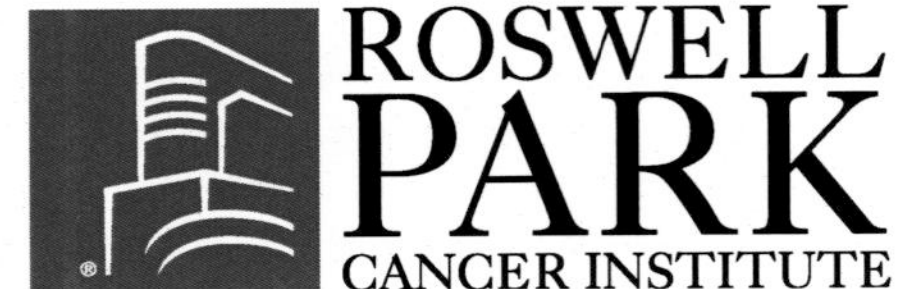

Established in 2007, the applied technology laboratory for advanced surgery program at Roswell Park Cancer Institute began as a safety and quality assurance initiative and has grown into a global training center for robot-assisted surgery. Our dedicated staff has helped many novice surgical teams establish safe robot-assisted surgical programs at their institutions across the globe. Our research program has designed and piloted several ground-breaking inventions which include one of the first robotic simulators and initiatives in artificial intelligence, patient safety and operating room communications.

Contributors

AUTHORS

Ahmed Aly, MBBS
Bryan Wittmeyer, MS, PT
Carol DeNysschen, Ph.D, R.D., M.P.H., C.D.N.
Cathrin McMullin, RN, BSN, OCN
Erinn Field Perusich, MHA
Jennifer Hydeman, Ph.D.
Johar Syed, MD
Katherine Szymanski
Kathleen Field, RN
Kathleen O'Leary, MD
Katie Kulesz, LPN
Khurshid A. Guru, MD
Linda K. Leising, RD, CDN
Mary Platek, Ph.D.
Melissa Hiscock BSN, RN, CWOCN, OCN
R. Seiji Ohtake, B.Sc. (P.T.)
Seraaj Fayyaz
Shabnam Bashir, MD
Youssef Ahmed, MD

CONTENT EDITING

Amy Dickinson
Sue Banchich

DESIGN & ILLUSTRATION

Yana Hammond, CMI
Iman Carr

AKNOWLEDGEMENTS

Roswell Park Alliance Foundation

The Robert P. Huben Endowed
Professorship of Urologic Oncology

The Zimmer Family Fund

Index